Madness and Creativity in Literature and Culture

Madness and Creativity in Literature and Culture

Edited by

Corinne Saunders and Jane Macnaughton

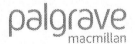

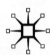

820.9
M182

First published 2005 by
PALGRAVE MACMILLAN
Houndmills, Basingstoke, Hampshire RG21 6XS and
175 Fifth Avenue, New York, N.Y. 10010
Companies and representatives throughout the world

PALGRAVE MACMILLAN is the global academic imprint of the Palgrave
Macmillan division of St. Martin's Press, LLC and of Palgrave Macmillan Ltd.
Macmillan® is a registered trademark in the United States, United Kingdom
and other countries. Palgrave is a registered trademark in the European
Union and other countries.

ISBN 1–4039–2199–7 hardback

This book is printed on paper suitable for recycling and made from fully
managed and sustained forest sources.

A catalogue record for this book is available from the British Library.

Library of Congress Cataloging-in-Publication Data
Madness and creativity in literature and culture / edited by Corrine
    Saunders and Jane Macnaughton.
        p. cm.
    Includes bibliographical references and index.
    ISBN 1–4039–2199–7
        1. English literature–History and criticism. 2. Psychoanalysis and
literature. 3. Mentally ill, Writings of the–History and criticism.
4. Authorship–Psychological aspects. 5. Literature–Psychological aspects.
6. Creation (Literary, artistic, etc.) 7. Authors, English–Psychology.
8. Literature and mental illness. 9. Mental illness in literature.
10. Mentally ill in literature. 11. Creative ability. I. Saunders, Corrine, 1963–
II. Macnaughton, Jane.

PR149.P78M33 2004
820.9'3561–dc22   2004053147

10   9   8   7   6   5   4   3   2
14   13   12   11   10   09   08   07   06   05

Printed and bound in Great Britain by
Antony Rowe Ltd, Chippenham and Eastbourne

To David Fuller and Andrew Russell
and to the memory of Roy Porter

Contents

Part III   Writing Madness: Psychoanalysis and Literature

List of Illustrations

Acknowledgements

The essays in this volume are all based on lectures given for the Public Lecture Series *Madness and Creativity: The Mind, Literature and Medicine,* held at the University of Durham between 2001 and 2002. We should like to thank the Vice-Chancellor, Sir Kenneth Calman, for his interest and support, and the University of Durham Public Lectures Fund and Centre for Arts and Health in Humanities and Medicine for their generous contributions to the costs of the lecture series. We are especially grateful to the Wellcome Trust for a grant towards the series. David Fuller would like to acknowledge the generous support of the British Academy in financing attendance at the conference 'Blake in the Orient' (Kyoto University, November 2003), organised by Professor Masashi Suzuki and Dr Steve Clark, to present an earlier version of his essay, 'Madness as "Other"'. A Research Leave Award from the Arts and Humanities Research Board allowed Corinne Saunders to complete the editing of the volume. We are grateful too to the Department of English Studies for their support, and to the participants and audiences of the lectures for their stimulating contributions and discussion.

We have incurred many other debts in the making of the book. The editors and production staff of Palgrave Macmillan have been unfailingly helpful. David Fuller generously transcribed the two dialogues and the essay of Roy Porter. We are especially grateful to Natsu Hattori for permission to print Roy's essay after his untimely death. We dedicate the volume to the memory of Roy Porter, whose work has so much defined the discipline of medical history and the study of madness and literature. We dedicate it also to David Fuller and Andrew Russell, in thanks for their constant encouragement, interest and support.

Notes on Contributors

Al Alvarez has played a prominent role in British literary culture since the 1950's, as poet, critic and writer. For ten years he was poetry critic and editor for the *Observer*, introducing American poets such as Lowell, Berryman and Plath, as well as Eastern European poets; he published the influential anthology *The New Poetry* in 1962. His many other publications include a celebrated study of suicide, *The Savage God* (1971); *Life After Marriage: Scenes from a Divorce* (1982); *Night: Night Life, Night Language, Sleep and Dreams* (1995); studies of Donne (1961) and Beckett (1973); several volumes of poetry, including *Autumn to Autumn and Selected Poems, 1953–1976* (1978); three novels; and an autobiography, *Where Did It All Go Right?* (1999).

Pat Barker is best known for her acclaimed trilogy of novels on the First World War, *The Regeneration Trilogy* (1996). Her own roots in the North-East inform her first novel, *Union Street* (1982), which focuses on the poverty associated with failing industry in this area in the 1970's. Her other novels include *Blow Your House Down* (1984), *The Century's Daughter* (1986) and *The Man Who Wasn't There* (1989). Most recently she has published the best-selling *Border Crossing* (2001) which is currently being adapted for film, and *Double Vision* (2002).

A. S. Byatt is both writer and literary critic. Her numerous works of fiction include *Possession*, for which she won the Booker Prize (1990), *Shadow of a Sun* (1964), *The Game* (1967), *The Virgin in the Garden* (1978), *Still Life* (1985), *Sugar and Other Stories* (1987), *Angels and Insects* (1991), and *The Biographer's Tale* (2000). Her critical works include a study of Wordsworth and Coleridge, *Unruly Times* (1970), a study of Iris Murdoch, *Degrees of Freedom* (1994), and two collections of essays, *Passions of the Mind* (1991) and *On Histories and Stories* (2000).

Robin Downie is Professor of Moral Philosophy at the University of Glasgow. He has an interest in teaching and writing in the areas in which medicine and the humanities overlap: ethics, literature and the arts. He has collaborated with Sir Kenneth Calman in writing *Healthy Respect: Ethics in Health Care* (1987) and with Dr Jane Macnaughton in writing *Clinical Judgement: Evidence in Practice* (2000).

Martyn Evans is at the forefront of the new interdisciplinary field of medical humanities. After a number of years at the University of Swansea, he has recently taken up the new Chair of Humanities in Medicine at the

University of Durham, one of only three chairs in the discipline in the UK. He is involved with the new School for Health and the Centre for the Arts and Humanities in Health and Medicine at Durham. He teaches philosophy and ethics of health care, and contributed to the design and teaching of Britain's first MA in Medical Humanities. He is founding co-editor of the journal *Medical Humanities*. He has published on the philosophy of music, research ethics, the definition of human death, organ transplantation, philosophy of medicine and the scope of medical humanities. His current research interests concern the role of the humanities in medical education and our understanding of medicine's nature and goals.

David Fuller is Professor of English Studies in the University of Durham. He has researched and written on a wide range of topics from the Renaissance to the Modern periods. He has particular interests in poetry, religion and music, and has worked extensively on William Blake. He is the author of *Blake's Heroic Argument* (1988), *James Joyce's 'Ulysses'* (1992), and, with David Brown, *Signs of Grace* (1995). He has also edited Marlowe's *Tamburlaine the Great* (1998), Blake's poetry for the Longman Annotated Texts series (2000), and, with Patricia Waugh, *The Arts and Sciences of Criticism* (1999). His current research is on reading poetry aloud.

Allan Ingram is Professor of English and Head of the Centre for Humanities Research at the University of Northumbria at Newcastle. His principal publications include *Boswell's Creative Gloom* (1982), *Intricate Laughter in the Satire of Swift and Pope* (1986) and *The Madhouse of Language* (1991), as well as two editions of eighteenth-century mad and medical writing, *Voices of Madness* (1997) and *Patterns of Madness in the Eighteenth Century* (1998). He is currently completing a monograph on eighteenth-century representations of insanity.

Jane Macnaughton is a general practitioner and Director of the Centre for Arts and Humanities in Health and Medicine at the University of Durham. She teaches personal and professional development to undergraduate medical students. She co-authored the book, *Clinical Judgement* (2000), with Robin Downie, another contributor to this volume, and has published papers on medical education, medical humanities, history of medicine and arts in health. Her current research is on the notion of hospitals as a cultural resource and is based on an empirical study of public engagement with an arts in hospital project.

Michael O'Donnell is well known as a doctor, writer and broadcaster. He has made many contributions to Radio 4, notably as chairman of the series *My Word* with Frank Muir and Dennis Norden, and has written and presented more than 90 TV programmes in Europe and the US. He was editor of

World Medicine for 15 years and has written regular columns for *The Times*, *The Guardian* and *Vogue*. He is the author of two novels and a number of books about medicine, including *A Sceptic's Medical Dictionary* (1997).

Michael O'Neill is Professor and Chairman of English Studies in the University of Durham. His extensive publications in the field of Romanticism include *The Human Mind's Imaginings: Conflict and Achievement in Shelley's Poetry* (1989), *Percy Bysshe Shelley: A Literary Life* (1989), and *Romanticism and the Self-Conscious Poem* (1997). He has edited a collection of essays on Shelley for the Longman Critical Readers series (1993), and is co-editing Shelley for the Oxford Authors Series. His other major research interest is in poetry of the 1930s and the post-war period. He is the author of numerous essays in this area, and, with Gareth Reeves, of *Auden, MacNeice, Spender: The Thirties Poetry* (1992). He is a poet himself: his collection *The Stripped Bed* (1990) won a prestigious Cholmondeley award.

Adam Piette is Reader in English at Glasgow University. Dr Piette's publications include *Remembering and the Sound of Words* (1996) and *Imagination at War* (1995), a study of fiction and poetry from 1939–1944.

Roy Porter was one of the leading and founding scholars in the new field of medicine and literature: his death in March, 2002 deprived the intellectual community of a remarkable authority. He stood out among his generation as a medical historian, both for his pioneering and acclaimed academic work and for his immensely prolific nature – he published more than 80 books and many articles. He was until 2001 professor in the Wellcome Trust Institute for the History of Medicine at University College London. One of his particular interests was the history of psychiatry, and just before he died, he published *Madness: A Brief History*, a work that considers perceptions of madness from the classical period to the twentieth century.

Corinne Saunders is Reader in the Department of English Studies at the University of Durham. She specialises in medieval literature and the history of ideas. She has particular interests in the history of women and in the history of medicine. Her publications include *The Forest of Medieval Romance* (1993), *Rape and Ravishment in the Literature of Medieval England* (2001), a Blackwell Critical Guide to *Chaucer* (2001), and a *Companion to Romance* (2004), which considers the transformations of the genre from its classical origins to the present. She is also working on a study of *Magic in Medieval Romance*.

Ignês Sodré is a psychoanalyst with a particular interest in literature, theories of literary creativity, and the human need for stories, comparable to the need to dream. She has written various papers on literature, in particular on George Eliot. With A. S. Byatt she has published a study of the creative process, *Imagining Characters: Six Conversations about Women Writers* (ed. Rebecca Swift, Chatto, 1995), which also takes the form of a dialogue.

Stephen Sykes is Professor of Theology in the University of Durham and Principal of St John's College, Durham; he was formerly Bishop of Ely, Regius Professor of Divinity in the University of Cambridge, and Van Mildert Professor in the University of Durham. He is Chair of the Church of England Doctrine Commission, and of the Inter-Anglican Theological and Doctrinal Commission. He has written extensively on modern theology and Anglicanism, and has special interests in mental health and medical ethics, as well as in William Cowper. His many works include *Christian Theology Today* (1971), *The Identity of Christianity* (1984), *Unashamed Anglicanism* (1995), and *The Story of Atonement* (1997).

Patricia Waugh is Professor of English Studies in the University of Durham. Her extensive publications in the areas of intellectual history, critical theory and modern fiction include *Metafiction: The Theory and Practice of Self-Conscious Fiction* (1984); *Feminine Fictions: Revisiting the Postmodern* (1989); *Practising Postmodernism: Reading Modernism* (1992); *The Harvest of the Sixties: English Literature and its Backgrounds 1960–90* (1995); and *Revolutions of the Word: Intellectual Contexts for the Study of Modern Literature* (1997). She has also edited a number of works, including (with David Fuller) *The Arts and Sciences of Criticism* (1999). She is currently completing a study of science and art in writings on utopia and the ideal moral commonwealth.

Introduction

Corinne Saunders and Jane Macnaughton

And all who heard should see him there,
And all should cry, Beware! Beware!
His flashing eyes, his floating hair!
Weave a circle round him thrice,
And close your eyes with holy dread,
For he on honey-dew hath fed,
And drunk the milk of Paradise.
(Samuel Taylor Coleridge, 'Kubla Khan')

O the mind, mind has mountains; cliffs of fall
Frightful, sheer, no-man-fathomed. Hold them cheap
May who ne'er hung there. Nor does long our small
Durance deal with that steep or deep. Here! Creep,
Wretch, under a comfort serves in a whirlwind: all
Life death does end and each day dies with sleep.
(Gerard Manley Hopkins, 'No worst, there is none')

Madness is one of the great topoi of literature from the classical period onwards. In part, this reflects the fearful yet compelling power of the idea of madness in western culture more generally. Mental illness, a terrible reality for some, is recognised by all. 'O, let me not be mad, not mad, sweet heaven! / Keep me in temper. I would not be mad' says Shakespeare's King Lear – and whether it is voiced or not, perhaps that sentiment is universal.[1] The darkness and disorder of the mind offer writers subjects of enduring interest precisely for their dreadful fascination. They provide some of the most powerful images of social disorder and of individual disintegration. Who can forget the suicide of Ophelia, the descent of Othello into madness, or the gradual overturning of the mind of Lady Macbeth? Against such violent fragmentation of the self, medicine can too often seem useless: 'Canst thou not minister to a mind diseased?' demands Macbeth of the physician, who can reply only, 'Therein the patient must minister to

1

himself'.[2] Earlier in the play, the doctor's words to the gentlewoman who watches with him as Lady Macbeth sleepwalks recall what is often the only resort beyond the self, 'More needs she the divine than the physician'.[3] Yet madness has another side: in its very darkness, illumination may be found. Thus Lear learns in and through his madness that whatever his status, 'unaccommodated man is no more but such a poor bare, forked animal', and ultimately, that love cannot be constrained.[4] The assumed madness of Hamlet allows him to seek the truth of Claudius' guilt, but also draws him deep into existential questions and into a cycle of destruction that blurs the boundaries between madness and sanity. The paradoxical association of mental disorder with self-knowledge recurs across western writing, and is linked to the possibility that writing, and art more generally, may be produced through the experience of illness or 'madness'. Madness and creativity have traditionally been connected: in ancient ideas of the poetic frenzy of the rhapsode, in the figure of the prophet, in the myth of the mad artist, in the notion of the writing cure, and in a long tradition of writing from as well as about the disorder of the mind. Madness has provided a literary subject since the classical period, while writers as various as Thomas Hoccleve in the medieval period, William Cowper in the eighteenth century, and Virginia Woolf and Sylvia Plath in the twentieth all experience some kind of mental disorder or 'madness' that not only shapes their writing but also inspires particular literary works – though that experience, as the contrast between Coleridge's description of the wild visionary and Hopkins' 'terrible sonnet' that maps his own despair suggests, may be anguished rather than romantic. This volume traces, explores and probes the sometimes uneasy, sometimes fascinating, always compelling relation between madness and creativity in writing and in culture.

The stimulus for this book was the founding at the University of Durham in 2000 of a Centre for Arts and Humanities in Health and Medicine. The Centre's function, of bringing together the disciplines of the Arts and Humanities with those of Health and Medicine, was described by Sir Kenneth Calman, the Vice-Chancellor of the University, as 'an idea whose time has come'. The Centre is engaged in research and education in two emerging fields, that of the Arts in therapeutic practice and community health and development, and that of Medical Humanities. Medical Humanities involves both the study of the arts in medicine – how literature, philosophy, history, music and art can inform and enlighten medical practice and doctors' understanding of the human condition – and the study of medicine in the arts, including the literary portrayal and function of aspects of medicine and illness, history of medicine, psychoanalytic theory, and the connection between illness and creativity.

One of the launch ventures of the Centre for Arts and Humanities in Health and Medicine was a major collaborative project with the Department of English Studies at the University of Durham, a public lecture series on 'The Mind, Medicine and Literature: Madness and Creativity'. The aim of the series was to promote research into the relationship between literature and medicine – and by extension, illness. The lectures, held in the autumn of 2001 and spring of 2002, offered the perspectives of academics, writers and medics, and included speakers from both within and without the University. The interests of contributors spanned classical to modern literature, and the academic emphasis was complemented by the practical insights of physicians and the creative insights of writers. The series provided the basis for this collection of essays.

Like the lecture series, this volume places particular emphasis on changing attitudes to madness reflected in literature, and explores the relationship between mental illness and creativity as it is represented in English literature from medieval to modern times. Essays consider the treatment and function of madness in writing across a range of English authors, in particular, poets. They draw special attention to the connection between 'madness' and writing, most obvious in groups of poets such as Christopher Smart, William Cowper, William Blake and John Clare, and Robert Lowell, John Berryman and Sylvia Plath, but evident from the Middle Ages onwards. Contributors explore the creative power of madness as literary topos, the ways mental illness may stimulate creative writing, the possibility of writing as therapy and the kinds of writing that are produced through the experience of mental illness. A particular focus is the recurrent association of 'madness', religious epiphany and writing.

The essays span the interrelated subjects of the mind, specifically the state of 'madness' or mental illness; medicine, in particular attitudes to and the treatment of mental illness; and literature, both as representing the experience of madness and cultural responses to it, and as produced through the state of 'madness' or recovery, a process that may itself become a literary subject. In part, the focus is historical. The collection as a whole illuminates the history of medicine: various essays demonstrate the shifts and continuities in clinical understandings of and social attitudes to mental illness from the Middle Ages, through the 'enlightened' notions of the eighteenth century, to the development of psychoanalysis and contemporary clinical approaches. As Michel Foucault has shown, the treatment of mental illness may be seen to mirror cultural ideologies. Literature, however, may provide alternative perspectives, and may set against the notions of asylum and confinement an interest in probing the state of the mind and the nature of mental illness as a fundamental aspect of the human condition.

It might be argued that the subject of this volume, which seeks to bring together medicine and literature, was almost inescapable given the fascination of writers with the subject of madness and the medical profession's quandary over the treatment of a set of conditions that seem to give rise to extraordinary creativity. From a clinical perspective, it was not the aim of the series to examine the biochemical, neurophysiological or even psychological abnormalities that might contribute to psychotic illness. Rather, a central aim was to reflect upon how doctors can learn about those who suffer such illness from those who have written creatively about it, either from the perspective of personal experience or imaginative understanding.[5] Some doctors, such as Anthony Storr and Kay Redfield Jamison, have themselves written about the association between madness and the artistic temperament. Storr, in his book about the relationship between solitariness and creativity, reports a number of studies that suggest a link between creativity and psychiatric illness, particularly depression.[6] He argues that this link is no accident,

> ... that the creative process can be a way of protecting the individual against being overwhelmed by depression; a means of regaining a sense of mastery in those who have lost it, and, to a varying extent, a way of repairing the self damaged by bereavement or by the loss of confidence in human relationships which accompanies depression from whatever cause.[7]

Jamison, herself a sufferer from manic depressive psychosis, also writes about the benefits of madness. She describes the experience of hypomania in this way:

> When you're high it's tremendous. The ideas and feelings are fast and frequent like shooting stars, and you follow them until you find better and brighter ones. Shyness goes, the right words and gestures are suddenly there, the power to captivate others a felt certainty. There are interests found in uninteresting people. Sensuality is pervasive and the desire to seduce and be seduced irresistible. Feelings of ease, intensity, power, well-being, financial omnipotence, and euphoria pervade one's marrow.[8]

It is possible instinctively to understand why such an experience might lead to creativity, but Daniel Nettle, as a psychologist, breaks the association down. Firstly, he says, hypomania facilitates the speed and range of the imagination. Secondly, the hypomanic becomes very energetic and driven even when what he or she is doing does not appear to offer any immediate benefit. And thirdly, despite this apparent lack of reward, the hypomanic experiences a feeling of extraordinary self belief that he or she is able to achieve great and difficult things which will be of benefit or interest to others.[9]

Thus madness can itself be like a drug that allows the sufferer to experience a kind of creative 'high'. So seductive is this state that even Jamison herself, despite fully understanding the consequences of non-compliance, admits to a deep reluctance to take medication.[10] This collection of essays illustrates some of the potential results of the creative 'high' but also raises questions about whether art can truly stem from a process that ultimately leads to chaos and disorder. The empowering surge of creative genius felt by the hypomanic soon tips over into mania and down to depression:

> The fast ideas are too fast, and there are far too many of them; overwhelming confusion replaces clarity. Memory goes. Humor and absorption on friends faces are replaced by fear and concern. Everything previously moving with the grain is now against – you are irritable, angry, frightened, uncontrollable, and enmeshed totally in the blackest caves of the mind.[11]

And so, while the following essays give some credence to the romantic idea of madness as a price worth paying for the creative muse, this view is balanced by accounts of the sufferings of the mentally ill and by the assertion that chaotic and disordered thinking may also be the enemy of great art.

Underpinning the collection, then, is the concept of a dialogue between medicine and literature: while literature finds a subject in and may be produced through mental illness, it is also the case that literature may provide new ways into the medical understanding of such illness. The first group of essays focuses on this aspect of the subject. Contemporary medicine, and particularly psychotherapy, emphasise the need for humane 'narrative understanding' of case histories as well as for the detached classification of symptoms. The study of 'story' and interpretation has entered the medical curriculum, accompanied by a new awareness of the psychological and ethical insights offered by literary portrayals of illness. Medicine may be seen as having creative or 'performative' aspects and the patient-medic dialogue as 'narrative'.

The volume as a whole, and in particular this first section, illustrates the power both of writing triggered by the actual experience of madness and of writing inspired by imaginative understanding of that experience. Doctors can learn to appreciate the pain of Cowper, who wrote during a period of insanity, 'I, fed with judgment, in a fleshy tomb, am / Buried above ground'.[12] But clinicians can also learn from writers such as A. S. Byatt, who explains how she entered into the mind of her protagonist to write about his horrific dream, 'I threw myself into this dream as a writer by in a sense dreaming it'.[13] The imaginative empathy in which the writer is engaged acts as an example for doctors who must develop this same sense of empathetic understanding of their patients.

Jean Dominique Bauby's moving account of his personal experience of 'locked in syndrome' has become a classic work for medical students learning about illness through literature.[14] He became completely paralysed following a brain stem stroke but was able to dictate the entire book letter by letter by blinking his left eye in response to repeated recitation of the alphabet by his interpreter. The shocking revelation of an active mind behind an immobile body challenges the assumptions clinicians may make about patients purely on the basis of their appearance. While 'locked-in syndrome' of this physical kind might give rise to madness if not recognised, no less moving is the fictional account of a similar experience brought about by psychological damage in Paul Sayer's book, *The Comforts of Madness*.[15] The narrator, Peter, tells of his breakdown while attempting suicide. An unwelcome saviour finds him by the edge of the sea:

> But his helping hands had to take all my weight. I could not move, had no strength, no desire to. Nothing was left in me at all. He laid me back on the hot sand and I reflected on the first wave of a warm, comforting stillness breaking over me, a quiet madness of my own making. In a funny sort of way it was how I imagined a homecoming might be.[16]

Such an account elicits from the reader an emotional response, enabling us to understand Peter's feeling of relief at withdrawing so dramatically from physical interaction with the world around him. This response is unlike any elicited by a dry, clinical case history, which may give the facts of the illness but does not convey the feeling. The facts are essential but the feeling is what makes the relationship between doctor and patient effective and, indeed, therapeutic. Real feeling, real understanding, genuine responses are crucial to the development of a trusting, therapeutic relationship with patients, whatever their diagnosis. Literature and drama enable clinicians to experience what madness is like and to understand more fully the pain of their patients. Insights from writing about madness and by the mentally ill are, therefore, increasingly drawn on in the education of doctors and medical students. Medicine has drawn fresh attention to the importance and multi-faceted quality of madness as a literary subject.

The second group of essays focuses on differing treatments and functions of madness in literature. Madness can become a key to human extremes and to the nature of the mind, but can also serve to illuminate social attitudes – as, for instance, in Blake's characterisation of Bedlam as 'dens of despair' rather than 'house of bread', or Woolf's sharply ironic depiction of psychiatry. Madness may also play a symbolic role: writers as diverse as Shakespeare, Blake, Eliot and Mann employ the image of fragmentation of the mind to reflect the disease or degeneration of society, while the figure of the hysteric or 'madwoman in the attic' common in nineteenth-century writing offers a different kind of emblem of repressive cultural assumptions and gender stereotypes.

Madness is not necessarily portrayed as entirely negative: it can be connected with unusual understanding, or with the anguish endemic to the human condition, particularly through an experience such as war. Medieval and Renaissance thought classify love as a madness, a heightened state with both physical and mental symptoms of illness. Madness can also trigger the process of self-realisation – often linked to recognition of human frailty and sinfulness, as with the figure of Nebuchadnezzar, whose madness and repentance form recurrent literary subjects. Madness is ambiguous, both a state of disorder and opening onto some sort of heightened understanding. Literature is full of instances of self-realisation in illness, often mental illness, for which the sickroom and sickbed, and sometimes the asylum, provide archetypal settings: Mann's *The Magic Mountain* offers a powerful example. The association of madness and creativity is rooted in this connection of mental disorder and understanding.

Frequently, however, literature engages with the writer's own experience, and it is here that the relation of madness and creativity becomes most complex. The voices of writers, and especially poets, who have themselves suffered some form of mental breakdown recur across the collection. Michel Foucault's notion of the 'lyric glow of illness' is borne out from the Middle Ages onwards – though the relation of the writer to his or her illness is not always so easy as the term 'lyric' may suggest. Thus the fifteenth-century poet Hoccleve recounts his mental 'infirmity' and recovery in order to defend his sanity; Cowper, Clare and Hopkins write from the depths of despair; Lowell, Berrryman and Plath turn 'personal anguish into art'; the poetry of both Eliot and Pound engages in different ways with their experiences of breakdown and mental hospitals. Poetry finds much of its power in the extraordinary tension between the formal structures of literary art and the disorder of madness as explicit or implicit subject. Writers may be shaped by or look back on 'madness' of different kinds: Virginia Woolf offers a striking example of a novelist acutely informed by mental breakdown.

It is evident from the writing of, for instance, Hoccleve and Cowper, and, in a different way, Blake, that the experience of religion often plays a crucial role in the writer's understanding of mental suffering. The effect of extreme melancholia may be that the sufferer perceives himself as deeply sinful, and /or 'madness' may be understood as a manifestation of God's punishment; it may cause or be caused by loss of faith – yet religion may also provide a way out, by offering both a means of structuring experience and a more optimistic perspective in which God's mercy is available to 'the Castaway'. The creative process of religious understanding can take an epiphanic or visionary form, evident in the experiences of medieval mystics: sometimes, as in the cases of Julian of Norwich and Margery Kempe, this is triggered by illness; sometimes, as in the visionary poetry of Blake, its extremity can appear 'mad'. The collection demonstrates the unsatisfactory nature of employing the term 'religious mania' to explain the intricate relation of the experiences of mental illness and faith.

Is it possible to analyse further the relation between madness and creativity? A number of essays look back to the classical notion of poetic inspiration as madness or divine frenzy, an idea still resonant in western thought, and to the mysterious nature of inspiration, a force beyond the rational. The third group of essays considers writing through the lens of twentieth-century psychoanalytical theories of madness and creativity, which in many ways developed these classical ideas. Psychoanalytical theories based on Edmund Wilson's 'the wound and the bow' thesis of inspiration (the need for the wound of madness to create the magical bow of art) are tested in the context of modern fiction and contemporary, often reductionist, scientific theory. The common societal and artistic expectation of creative madness, 'the myth of the artist', may both inform and be challenged by imaginative writing. In this final section, the topic of how literature engages with and is inspired by the subject of madness is considered by writers themselves, in terms both of reading and writing. A particular interest is the distinction between fantasy and reality, and the contrast between the controlled writer and the 'mad' subject. Questions arise too of how biography, history, psychoanalytical theory and fiction interrelate. These essays illuminate the creative process from a writerly point of view, both in terms of 'writing madness' and of the intricate and highly problematic relation of madness and creativity as it is perceived and experienced.

In the opening essay of this volume, Roy Porter brings together literature and medicine by examining recent debates regarding the definition and treatment of insanity, focusing in particular on the need for a 'thick history' of psychiatry of a demystifying kind. His particular emphasis is the tension between the urge to understand the words of the mentally ill themselves and the Freudian impetus towards 'systematic distrust', the classification of speech as symptom rather than communication. He illustrates this theme with eyewitness accounts of both patients and those treating them, and considers too the shift from the notion of madness as sent by God to the notion of clinical illness. Attention is drawn to the large amount of extant writing by and about the mentally ill – literary, legal and autobiographical – and the neglect of this by historians. Porter draws on a wide range of works written by those who might be classified as mentally ill, often in counterpoint to psychoanalysis, to suggest sometimes provocative new ways of reading cases through attentiveness to the actual experiences and words of the patient, and in terms of cultural commentary. The madman, he argues, is always speaking, but is not always listened to – his words are reduced to symptomatic sound.

Michael O'Donnell continues Porter's theme of communication, focusing minutely on the relation between doctor and patient, this time from the point of view of the physician, to argue that creativity is an essential part of medical success, just as it is for the actor. The skill of the actor echoes that of the writer in that it enables viewers to understand the complex problems of the human condition: intense imaginative engagement with a subject in turn provokes a genuine emotional response. In the same way, the delicate relationship between doctor and patient elicits the narrative of illness, and allows for successful diagnosis. Like Porter, O'Donnell demonstrates the dangers of simple classification of words as symptoms, and the detrimental effects of negative communication. He thus challenges the typical boundaries between doctor or analyst and patient, and between health and illness – and further, emphasises the difference between notions of illness and disease. O'Donnell points to the ways that sophisticated literary comprehension of text and performance may enhance holistic medical analysis of illness, as well as to the practice of clinical skills by writers in their creation of a psyche. The study of literature and medicine allows for a return to the idea of medicine as 'the healing art'.

For Robin Downie too, creative writing offers an imaginative way into illness, and particularly madness, and complements the understandings of psychiatrists or scientists. Downie's essay probes the different ways in which madness may function in literature – either to advance the understanding of madness *per se*, or as a device or theme that enhances and reflects the literary work itself. Downie looks back to Plato to make a distinction similar to those of Porter and O'Donnell, between the scientific model, which aims at classification by tracing recurrent patterns in mental disorder, and the literary model, which puts events within a sequence or context in order to create narrative understanding. Downie's central example is Virginia Woolf's portrayal of Septimus Smith's madness in *Mrs Dalloway*, a particularly powerful instance in light of Woolf's own mental illness and her experience of psychiatry in the 1920's. Downie contrasts such attempts to promote the understanding of human psychology with the potentially inhibiting use of mad stereotypes such as that of Mrs Rochester in *Jane Eyre* – a use redressed by Jean Rhys in *Wide Sargasso Sea*, where the focus is Antoinette / Bertha's own psyche.

As Downie's essay suggests, madness plays a prominent role in writing from the classical period through the Middle Ages to the present day. Corinne Saunders considers the treatment of madness in some of the earliest writings in English, to show both striking contrasts with post-Freudian understandings of mental illness and some notable continuities. Medieval attitudes to madness were profoundly different in that the mad were in general not shut away; madness was seen as sent by God, a mysterious part of his providential patterning, although there were also lively medical and legal discourses of madness. Saunders sets these against medieval literary texts, which frequently characterise madness as a reversion to bestiality and as a punishment for sin. This lack of control also has a more positive side, however, in the prominent theme of love-malady, so masterfully employed by Chaucer in *Troilus and Criseyde*. This secular notion finds its complement in the idea of mystical vision so powerful in medieval religious writing. As Roy Porter suggests, in modern terms the mystics may well be seen as exhibiting the symptoms of mental illness: it is precisely their distance from the everyday world, often manifested in physical illness, that opens the way to their visionary experience, and subsequently to the process of writing. An interesting contrast is found in the poetry of Thomas Hoccleve, the first writer in English to document descent into mental illness and recovery. Through Hoccleve's narrative we are made acutely aware of the silencing as well as the creative aspect of madness.

Allan Ingram continues the exploration of writing madness by examining the narratives of three eighteenth-century writers, all of whom experienced forms of mental illness: the diaries of James Boswell; the little-known account of depression written by a young widow, Hannah Allen; and the poems of Anne Finch. Ingram considers the expression of depression, the acknowledgement or confession of it, and the complex relation between experience and writing. As in the case of medieval understandings of madness, the perspectives of these writers are powerfully shaped by their religious belief, but what is striking is that their expression of the trouble of the mind goes far beyond the simple and submissive acceptance of affliction. Ingram demonstrates how Boswell's diaries are pervaded by his experience of illness, but also how compulsive telling, particularly of his sexual exploits, marks his mental state. Boswell's writings reflect a tension between the notions of writing as therapeutic and as indulgence of despair, and it is telling that at its height Boswell's depression was expressed only in silence. Hannah Allen's account of her depression is more constricted, but equally intense. Allen interprets her illness as sent by God, yet what is compelling is not her didactic interpretation, but the account of her mental disorder and the existential questions to which it leads, the testing of her faith. Anne Finch's poems offer a more conscious negotiation of depression, finding their intensity in the dialogue between melancholy and joy. But in all these instances, as in the case of Hoccleve, depression is disabling as well as creative, at its height silencing even while, paradoxically, it provides moments of inspiration and a purpose to writing.

The paradox of melancholy – its disabling yet creative force – is nowhere more evident than in Stephen Sykes' subject, the poetry of William Cowper. As with the writers discussed by Allan Ingram, in particular Hannah Allen, for Cowper Christian faith plays a crucial and paradoxical role in the experience of madness. Stephen Sykes poses the difficult question of how to address the religious belief of the mentally ill, demonstrating the brutal nature of the rationalist approach, which reduces Cowper's experience to religious mania. Sykes demonstrates clearly the intermittent quality of Cowper's experience of what were probably episodes of manic depression, drawing on contemporary psychiatric research as well as Cowper's autobiography and letters. In probing the sense fundamental to Cowper's melancholy of having committed an unforgivable sin, Sykes combats the easy association of this with Calvinistic notions of sin and judgement, and election to grace, showing the complexity, balance and potential for grace through contrition in the moderate brand of Calvinism espoused by John Newton, Cowper's close friend and theological confidant. It is Cowper's own mental affliction that underlies his religious crisis and terrible sense of abandonment by God. The late poem 'The Castaway', telling of a sailor washed overboard and left to drown, becomes a tragic emblem of Cowper's situation, and functions too as a call to those in whom he trusts to provide some hope of rescue and spiritual encouragement. Sykes draws on Cowper's writings and their contexts to compare their dialogue between despair and hope with the Biblical dialectic of affirmation and negation. For Cowper, Sykes argues, writing becomes a means of negotiating the deep paradoxes of faith of which his illness made him so acutely aware, and until near the end of his life provided him with a means of containing melancholy.

For Cowper, madness was a deep and life-long affliction, formative and devastating. David Fuller probes a very different relation of madness and poetry in his consideration of William Blake. He begins with Blake's annotation of Spurzheim's observations on insanity: Blake recounts how Cowper visited him in spirit to tell him that he was 'mad as a refuge from unbelief – from Bacon, Newton and Locke', that is, as an antidote to rationalism. Blake repeatedly played on this notion of madness, which forms a recurrent theme in his writing and designs. Yet while Blake's visionary quality caused him to be placed as mad by numerous critics from the eighteenth century to the twentieth, Fuller demonstrates the credulity and irrationality inherent in taking Blake's madness literally. Blake rather recuperates madness, drawing as Renaissance writers did on classical notions of inspiration and the idea of genius: madness in his work functions as metaphor and condition, as an emblem of escape from the constriction of Enlightenment thought and of the necessary alienation of the artist. At the same time, Blake treats actual madness in a detached and sympathetic manner, not as a sufferer but as one sympathetic to the terrible abuses of Bedlam with its 'dens of despair' and to the incomprehensibility of mental illness. Fuller shows that Blake's own visionary experience is not characterised by simple enthusiasm or mental disorder, but by controlled, poised and intelligent writing, which engages at a profound level with the need for art to move the spirit, both of poet and reader. When Blake calls for 'madness' he calls for the engagement of the visionary imagination.

Michael O'Neill's essay explores further many of the ideas regarding madness and vision emerging from Fuller's discussion of Blake. O'Neill takes as his starting point Coleridge's notion, rooted in classical thought, that the hallmark of the imaginative poet is also the characteristic of a person in the grip of mania. This notion partly underlies the fact that 'madness' is a recurrent theme in both nineteenth- and twentieth-century poetry, and is often treated with startling empathy. Yet the relation of madness and poetry is also paradoxical, for writing about the experience of madness, even, for instance, John Clare's deeply personal asylum poems, tends to employ rigorous formal control. The tension between mental disorder and formal order, O'Neill argues, becomes a heightened version of the tension between experience and artifice evident in most poetry, and is well-exemplified by the eerie and beautiful lyrics in the medic-poet Thomas Beddoes' *Death's Jest Book*, which seems to speak from 'beyond' the madness/rationality divide. Browning, Shelley and Tennyson all treat the subject of mania, often as response to society. The sense of madness as protest is especially evident in twentieth-century poetry, for instance, in the writing of Yeats and Eliot. O'Neill ends with a consideration of Robert Lowell, John Berryman and Sylvia Plath, all of whose poetry engages with their own experiences of mental illness, though again often in relation to the disintegration of society. Here too, O'Neill demonstrates the extraordinary formal control, even impersonality, through which personal, mental anguish becomes art. The themes of alienation and disintegration move far beyond the simply confessional.

Martyn Evans' essay provides an important counterpoint to Fuller and O'Neill, by treating the themes of the mind, medicine and creativity in a novel, Thomas Mann's *The Magic Mountain*. Set in a mountain sanatorium for the sufferers of tuberculosis, the principal theme of the novel is illness. Evans reads the work to open out philosophical questions, in particular that of the relation of the mind and body in illness, a continuum also central to medieval mystical writing. Mann treats illness as a kind of mystical mental state, in which existential questions of life and death are illuminated, and which may also produce a dark creative force. In his own illness, the book's protagonist, Hans Castorp, like the mystics, courts knowledge by placing himself in extreme physical, mental and moral situations, in which he enters a state of feverish imagining, marked by both physical and mental symptoms. Like Blake and the poets treated by O'Neill, Mann is especially interested in the state of society, and the novel focuses in particular on the decadence of society, for which illness becomes a metaphor. In illness, Castorp, like his fellows, is fascinated by death, yet finally, through his series of visionary experiences of intellectual and moral darkness, he gains a sense of morality and hope. Set against Castorp are the caricatured figures of the Freudian psychoanalyst and the sanatorium's medical director, who places exclusive emphasis on the physical at the expense of the mental: suppression of the mind is ultimately shown to lead to madness. Yet, Evans argues, for Mann literary creation is ultimately situated within that intoxication and darkness associated with the drive to death, with the profane, the primeval, the disordered: in that sense creativity is itself a disease. The power of the novel, he suggests, lies not in Castorp's enlightenment but in its evocation of creative darkness.

Literature and psychoanalysis often enjoy an uneasy relationship. In her essay, Pat Waugh addresses some of the most fundamental questions regarding the association of madness and creativity for a (post)modern audience. Waugh shows how the twentieth century saw a revival of the myth of Dionysus, the classical notion of artistic madness (the wound) as God-like creativity (necessary to the magical bow of art). Waugh argues, however, that this revival is less a response of writers themselves than of psychoanalysts, critics and theorists, often in answer to the reductionism of science, of which she provides a series of powerful examples. Yet in actuality, the Dionysian myth shares some of this reductionism in its construction of reason as scientific rationality, against which all else is identified as madness. In particular, Waugh argues, the myth ignores the possibility of ethical choice: she challenges the readings of Freud, R. D. Laing and Edmund Wilson, showing how Euripides' *The Bacchae*, which contains the Dionysus episode, and Sophocles' *Philoctetes*, with its wound and bow motif, demonstrate the possibility of exercising reason as an ethical agency. Against psychoanalytical theories she sets examples from the work of Joseph Conrad and Thomas Mann, both of whom, as Evans has also shown in relation to Mann, demonstrate the dangers of creative degeneracy. Waugh returns finally to Virginia Woolf, also the subject of Downie, to explore Woolf's theory of a disciplined art far from Dionysian frenzy. As O'Neill has argued in relation to poetry, art, even when it engages with or is inspired by madness, involves detachment, even renunciation of the ego, and requires control as well as sympathy.

Al Alvarez's essay is closely related in theme and emphasis to that of Waugh. Alvarez in part offers a retrospective on his own seminal work, *The Savage God* (1971), which, as Waugh notes, employs precisely the myth of artistic madness: Dionysus *is* the savage god. Yet, Alvarez argues, the myth has been taken up and promoted, both by the media and by artists themselves, in ways that he did not envisage, ways that, as Waugh and O'Neill argue, ignore the crucial aspect of control in art. Society's response in itself provides a telling index of contemporary values and of the direction of art. Alvarez looks back to the complex interrelation of art and mental disturbance in the 1960's and 1970's, a feature of the new 'extremist art' espoused by Robert Lowell, John Berryman and Sylvia Plath. Like the painting of the abstract expressionists, he argues, their poetry was situated on the friable edge between the tolerable and intolerable, and found energy within their chaotic personal lives. Yet at the same time, as for Rothko or Pollock, precision and detail were crucial. Art such as this, written on the edge, is dangerous: it does not involve self-therapy but the probing of sickness, and in order to make art out of despair, strict inner resources are necessary. Alvarez argues that the frequent critical focus on the life of Sylvia Plath ignores the sardonic, witty and detached tone of her poems, the sense of living on the edge of despair, yet still retaining control. He demonstrates clearly both the energy and tension provided by the experience of mental illness, and the incapacitating, silencing quality of a complete descent into 'madness'.

The dialogue of A. S. Byatt and Ignès Sodré takes as its point of departure Freud's essay 'Creative Writers and Day-Dreaming', which argues that writers transform fantasising and wishful thinking into art, but that extreme fantasy also leads to neurosis or psychosis. Byatt and Sodré explore these ideas in relation to two narratives that portray and engage profoundly with fantasy so extreme that it may be interpreted as madness, yet are highly controlled. A primary question is the boundary between fantasising and 'madness', the possibility of neurosis or mental illness without clinical insanity. They take first the case of Flaubert's *Madame Bovary*, to probe the depiction of the unreality of Emma Bovary's inner mental life. While the novel comments on the terrible repressiveness of bourgeois life, it also shows the destructiveness of total detachment from reality. Byatt and Sodré take as their second example Thomas Mann's portrayal of Aschenbach in *Death in Venice*, exploring the ways in which Aschenbach's obsession with the boy Tadziu allows for the blocking out of reality: like Evans, they show that degeneration and fantasy are closely linked in Mann's writing, though creativity is also situated in fantasy. A key aspect of their discussion is Aschenbach's Dionysian dream, which for Byatt and Sodré marks his mental breakdown. They focus on the self-consciousness of Mann's use of this myth of the artist, which draws closely on Nietzsche's discussion of the myth in *The Birth of Tragedy from the Spirit of Music*, in order to illuminate the opposition of reason and passion. The final part of their discussion focuses on Byatt's own use of dream as opening onto the repressed part of the psyche in her novel *The Biographer's Tale*. Byatt's mode is that of realism as she recreates the effect of profound mental disturbance on dream, but she shows how her writing also draws on other literary models and more general cultural experience. Byatt and Sodré conclude by considering the situation of the writer herself, split between the imaginative participation in the experience of madness and the detached, disciplined control necessary to write it. The split between beauty and horror, they argue, empowers art precisely through its dangerous fascination.

The dialogue between Pat Barker and Adam Piette focuses on the relation between writing and mental trauma, in particular, the trauma effected by the experience of war, the subject of Barker's *Regeneration* trilogy. Barker points robustly to the absolute necessity for cold-bloodedness in the writer, despite the fact that the work may be underpinned and inspired by the intense experience of horror, the stuff of nightmare. Piette compares this to the idea of medicine's split face, and the need expressed by Barker's character, the psychologist Rivers, for an almost impossible division of the self between involvement and objectivity. For Barker, there is a kind of cruelty in the writer's coolness and use of craftsmanship on the subject matter of horror: like Byatt, she speaks of the danger of writing. She endorses Piette's identification of the common concern in her novels with violence and trauma, and her interest in these dark areas of the psyche. Barker and Piette consider the need to negotiate the haunting of the psyche through a delicate balance of remembering and forgetting – the balance pursued by Rivers in his practice of psychology and experimentation with theories of the nervous system. For Rivers, as in the Dionysian myth of the artist, the primitive, 'mad' level was the source of creativity, often revealed by dreams and symbols. Barker suggests that the writer too is experimenting with such theories in setting up a fictional world with its own rules, and creating extraordinary personalities with their own psychical hinterlands. Like Alvarez and Byatt, Barker argues that because writers are constantly testing the boundary between fiction and reality, they occupy a dangerous mental territory: they too need both to remember and to forget the secret, dark places they evoke. Madness, similarly, is seductive, a compelling subject, yet also a dangerous one in its power to consume as well as to inspire, to destroy as well as to create, to silence as well as to speak.

Notes

1 William Shakespeare, *The Tragedy of King Lear*, in *The Complete Works*, ed. Stanley Wells and Gary Taylor, The Oxford Shakespeare (Oxford, 1988), Act 1, scene 4, lines 45–46.
2 Shakespeare, *Macbeth*, in *Complete Works*, Act 5, scene 5, lines 42, 48.
3 Shakespeare, *Macbeth*, in *Complete Works*, Act 5, scene 1, line 71.
4 Shakespeare, *The Tragedy of King Lear*, in *Complete Works*, Act 3, scene 4, lines 100–102.
5 For an account of the different forms of madness and what is known about their underlying brain mechanisms see Daniel Nettle, *Strong Imagination: Madness, Creativity and Human Nature* (Oxford, 2001), Chapters 1–5.
6 Anthony Storr, *Solitude* (London, 1997), p. 142.
7 Storr, p. 143.
8 Kay Redfield Jamison, *An Unquiet Mind: A Memoir of Moods and Madness* (London, 1996), p. 67. For a further account of the relationship between the artistic temperament and manic-depressive illness see Jamison, *Touched with Fire* (New York, 1994).
9 See Nettle, pp. 152–154.
10 Jamison, *An Unquiet Mind*, pp. 98–103.
11 Jamison, *An Unquiet Mind*, p. 67.
12 William Cowper, 'Lines Written During a Period of Insanity', in *William Cowper*, ed. Michael Bruce, Everyman's Library (London, 1999), p. 3.
13 See A. S. Byatt and Ignês Sodre, 'On Writing Madness', in this volume, pp. 200–19.
14 Jean-Dominique Bauby, *The Diving-Bell and the Butterfly* (London, 1997).
15 Paul Sayer, *The Comforts of Madness* (London, 1988).
16 Sayer, p. 105.

Part I

Reading Madness:
Literature in Medicine

1

Madness and Creativity: Communication and Excommunication

Roy Porter

Roy Porter gave this lecture at the University of Durham in the summer of 2001, and later that year at the University of Newcastle, where it was recorded. The lecture was written as the basis of an essay for this volume, and as the inaugural lecture for the Public Lecture Series 'Madness and Creativity: The Mind, Medicine and Literature', held at the University of Durham in 2001–2002. Roy died before he was able to revise the lecture to appear in print, although as will be evident it was already in a highly finished form. We have removed some of the colloquialisms and mannerisms of oral presentation, added references to the works cited, and in some cases completed quotations; we have also added in parentheses some explanatory detail regarding two of the writers instanced. We would like to thank Natsu Hattori for her generosity in allowing us to print the lecture, and for her editorial assistance. We are also grateful to Allan Ingram and David Fuller for their advice and assistance. Any errors are, of course, our own.

In his introduction at the University of Newcastle, Roy took particular pleasure in a notice in the lecture theatre, which read 'In the bin and not on the floor', playing on its relevance as an alternative title, and using the phrase later in his lecture.

***

Psychiatry had taken a wrong turn, argued two distinguished British psychiatrists, Richard Hunter and Ida Macalpine, in 1974. It was they who wrote that splendid book, *George III and the Mad-Business*, which became the basis of Alan Bennett's play and film.[1] They argued:

> Today neurotic types are also postulated who react to adversity by developing neurosis. It is assumed that mental pathology derives from normal psychology and can be understood in terms of faulty inter- or intrapersonal relationships and corrected by re-education or psychoanalysis

of where the patient's emotional development went wrong. Despite all efforts which have gone into this approach and all the reams devoted to it, results have been meagre not to say inconclusive and contrast sharply with what medicine has given to psychiatry and which is added to year by year.

Why was this, they asked. The answer was simple to them. They said, 'Patients are victims of their brain rather than their mind. To reap the rewards of this medical approach, however, means a reorientation of psychiatry from listening to looking ... .'[2] And that is what I want to follow up in much of this essay: different approaches to psychiatry, to understanding madness, relating to looking and listening.

The call by Richard Hunter and Ida Macalpine for psychiatry to turn away from listening to the mentally ill did not stem from any inhumanity on their part. It was the logical consequence of their medical credo. Mental illness, they believed, was not 'psychogenic'.[3] Hence the cries and complaints of the insane were essentially side-effects. They were symptoms of distress, but not in themselves disease, nor even necessarily good clues to the nature of disease. You didn't understand the mad by understanding what they said. Neither was there a Freudian 'talking cure' for madness. For Hunter and Macalpine, psychiatry ought to be based upon a rigorous somatic foundation. Reality had a biological base. Illness was organic, and mental illness was mainly neurophysiological. The preoccupation of depth psychiatry, of analytical psychiatry, with the consciousness of patients, and above all their unconscious, was thus a dead end. Hunter and Macalpine were in a fine position to judge, because their early joint work had been ultra-orthodox in its Freudianism, and only later did they, as it were, see the light and change sides in the psychiatric debate. And they did so with all the zeal of neophytes.

As a historian, it's not for me, because I don't have the competence, to judge what it is that psychiatrists ought to be doing – whether they ought to be looking at or listening to mental illness. As a historian, however, I'd like to qualify Hunter and Macalpine's assumption that psychiatry has mistakenly spent its time listening to its clients, because when I, as a historian, read case histories, asylum records, psychiatric textbooks from the seventeenth century up to the present, what I find too often is what you could call dialogues of the deaf. Those who have been shut up – put 'in the bin' – have all too often been shut up in the other sense – or at least, nobody has actually attended to what they have said, except to put down their dislocated speech as a proof of their derangement. The history of psychiatry tells tales less of communication than of excommunication. Certainly that is what patients themselves have thought down the centuries. An instance is John Perceval, son of the assassinated British Prime Minister, Spencer Perceval, and author of an extraordinarily moving autobiographical narrative of what it's like to be mad, called *A Narrative of the Treatment Received by a Gentleman, during a State of Mental Derangement*, published in 1838, the year after Queen Victoria came to the throne, and possibly the most perceptive as well as the most poignant of autobiographical records of insanity. Around 1830 John Perceval converted to an extreme evangelical Protestant sect, which promised a kind of hotline to God. When the Almighty spoke to him, Perceval reported, 'The sounds I heard were at times beautiful in the extreme, resembling the Greek language... '; 'I was usually addressed in verse...'.[4] Soon he was being assailed by a veritable pandemonium of voices, demonic as well as divine, tormented by his head of fire: '... I heard voices without and within me, and sounds as of the clanking of iron, and the breathing of great forge bellows, and the force of flames'.[5] He was judged mad by his family, and confined to an asylum, the sole side-benefit of which was, for him, that 'Here I might hollo or sing as my spirits commanded'.[6] Nevertheless, he was to discover during his eighteen-month sojourn in these asylums that the medical superintendents and staff never listened to his requests, and barely, as he experienced it, addressed him as a human being. 'Men acted', he complained,

> as though my body, soul, and spirit were fairly given up to their control, to work their mischief and folly upon. My silence, I suppose, gave consent. I mean, that I was never told, such and such things we are going to do; we think it advisable to administer such and such medicine, in this or that manner; I was never asked, Do you want any thing? do you wish for, prefer any thing? have you any objection to this or to that?[7]

And this kind of ostracism had been inflicted upon him from his very entry into the asylum when (as he put it):

> Instead of my understanding being addressed and enlightened, and of my path being made as clear and plain as possible, in consideration of my confusion, I was committed, in really difficult and mysterious circumstances, calculated of themselves to confuse my mind, even if in a sane state, to unknown and untried hands; and I was placed amongst strangers, without introduction, explanation or exhortation.[8]

The word 'introduction' is quite interesting: he was a gentlemen; he would expect to be introduced. And he was treated throughout, he accused, 'as if I were a piece of furniture, an image of wood, incapable of desire as well as of judgement'. This routine refusal of the authorities to communicate with him, this systematic denial of his humanity, as he saw it, proved, he was convinced, therapeutically counter-productive. He wrote:

> I was not ... once addressed by argument, expostulation, or persuasion. The persons round me consulted, directed, chose, ordered, and force was

the unica and ultima ratio applied to me. If I were insane, in my resolution to be silent, because I was sure that neither of the doctors, or of my friends, would understand my motives, or give credit to facts they had not themselves experienced; they were surely no less insane who, because of my silence, forgot the use of their own tongues... .[9]

Experiences like Perceval's, of being ignored, of being reduced to a kind of non-person-status, have been registered in any number of accounts written by ex-patients of psychiatric institutions. For example, in an exposé edited by two British members of Parliament as recently as the 1950s and entitled *The Plea for the Silent* (it could have been called *The Plea for the Silenced*), one former inmate recalls her experience of unremitting ostracism in a mental institution, an experience all too common at that time:

> I was not allowed to write to my employers to notify them of my inability to continue my work, and I was not allowed to write to my best friend to tell her where to locate me. No reason was ever given for this breach of the rules....
>
> Apart from replying to questions, and providing me with food, the staff ignored me. There I lay, perfectly quietly in bed, without a soul to whom I could voice the awful terror which consumed me, and with no knowledge of the staff's next step. It appeared that I was expected to lie in bed all day long, with nothing whatever to do, but suffer from the shock of certification and my terror of the future.
>
> I thought that this technique must be a new method devised for the study of mental illness; but I was soon to learn that it appeared to be nothing but a callous belief that the insane do not suffer and that any problems they may express are bound to be 'imaginary'. I heard, with mounting horror, the attempts of other new patients to get their needs satisfied and their efforts to obtain information; and I noted the evasions of the staff. No-one ever seemed to be able to get a sensible reply to any question.
>
> ...
>
> 'Where there is no sense there is no feeling', was a favourite saying of these nurses.[10]

In short, these were Perceval's allegations of ostracism precisely repeated over a century later.

How do we explain this state of affairs? To some degree obviously it was a consequence of simple short-comings. Poor staff, under-funding, overloading produced the banal brutality typical of total institutions down the ages, be they mental institutions, or prisons, or whatever. But the sins are not just those of omission but those of commission too. They are expressive of positive psychiatric structures, of scientific priorities and policy choices. Until early modern times, many historians, including the guru of the psychiatric historians, Michel Foucault, have argued – and have argued with some, but not complete, plausibility – that mad people were allowed to mingle with the sane, in society. Lunatics in those days were, of course, noted for their irregularities of thought and speech. Nicholas Culpeper, of herbal fame, in the seventeenth century noted that of course you could tell the mad apart from the sane because they were 'Sometimes laughing, singing, then sad, fearful, rash, doating, crying out, threatning, skipping, leaping, then serious, etc'.[11] But the point is that in those days before the mad were systematically shut up, madness might be thought of as having something to say. Madness could be seen as speaking the language, perhaps of God, or sometimes the devil, or on occasions it could be the effusions of poetic genius. Erasmus's heroine, Folly, in *The Praise of Folly*, spoke wisdom: here was madness talking sense. And truth, the Bible said, poured from the mouths of babes and sucklings, and also fools and simpletons. The jesters of Shakespeare's plays, like the Fool in *King Lear*, or Feste in *Twelfth Night*, assumed an antic disposition. They turned words on their heads, they twisted their tongues, they outwitted logic itself and gave voice to dark truths that sane people thought it impolitic to speak at court. The later imposition of what Foucault called 'the great confinement', the large scale and systematic locking up of certified mad people in institutions, changed that. Mass sequestration in madhouses – and it steadily grew in the eighteenth and nineteenth centuries until in England in the mid-twentieth century there were some 150,000 people locked away, mainly involuntarily, in institutions – some half a million people in the United States of America – necessarily quashed any such dialogue between madness and reason. Or, as Foucault put it, it reduced such truths that madness had been supposed to speak to the status of unreason, to something purely negative and meaningless, 'it was in relation to unreason and to it alone that madness could be understood'.[12] Visiting an Irish lunatic asylum in the middle of the last century, the inspectors were button-holed by a certain inmate who levelled against the institution an accusation of theft. 'They took my language from me', he accused the authorities.[13]

This kind of institutional silencing, or soundproofing, was rationalised and reinforced by the infant discipline of psychiatry. From the scientific revolution of the seventeenth century onwards, influential currents in medicine – Cartesian ones if you like – modelled man essentially as a machine, material in nature, with a disembodied soul, and thus reduced the moods and complaints of disorderly people to secondary manifestations, equivalent to the squeaks and judderings of a car engine needing repair. Something was obviously wrong, but nothing significant was being said. Madness, or the cries of madness, the complaints of madness, were a bit like (if you like) a belch, or a fart. The decibels of madness were all hot air. There was nothing in them to listen to and decode. And, reinforcing such newly-dominant medical materialism, wider cultural trends were further conspiring from the mid-seventeenth century onwards to depreciate and to disqualify the voice of mad people. Time had been when, for example in the Renaissance, Platonism had said that truth was within the word, in a sort of biblical sense: 'In the beginning was the Word' (John 1: 1). It was charged with supernatural and magical qualities. In the Bible, Adam names the animals, or in Greek mythology, Apollo charms the animals with his poetry and his song. But the empiricism dictated by the philosophy of the scientific revolution – by Thomas Hobbes, and by John Locke, for example – and by Enlightenment empiricist philosophy – reduced meaning to a matter of conventional signs conventionally ordered. It prized fact over fiction. It prized number over rhetoric. It prized things over words. It prized analysis over expressiveness. In other words, it devalued the truth of words in themselves. The Augustan aesthetics, in the age of Alexander Pope and Jonathan Swift, put forward the idea – and this is from Alexander Pope's *Essay on Criticism* – that 'the *Sound* must seem an *Eccho* to the *Sense*': sense comes first, rhetoric is secondary.[14] It construes artists as more like craftsmen than like visionaries. Mad poets thus lost their licence to conjure with words, and the old Platonic trope of the divine fire, the *furor* which enabled the imagination to see truths beyond common-sense reason, was supremely parodied in Alexander Pope's satirical vision in his *Dunciad* of sick Grub Street versifiers and hacks, skulking in their Cave of Spleen, obsessed by what he called, dismissively and reductively, 'the power of noise'. Their poetry had just become a lot of noise. Jonathan Swift's garrulous anti-heroes, the unreliable narrators of *A Tale of a Tub* and *Gulliver's Travels*, are just windbags: they are compulsive digressers; they entirely lack any self-awareness. The hero, the narrator of *A Tale of a Tub*, expresses the hope that one day he will finally 'be able to write upon nothing'.

These new philosophies, these new aesthetics, cast suspicion upon the old claims for speech. This, of course, had a kind of socio-political dimension as well: there were certain sorts of speech that were increasingly regarded by the respectable, polite society of the eighteenth century as dangerous, as devilish, as diabolical. There was a war against oral, plebeian culture, against dialect, against rustic diction, against the old habits of cursing and riddling, casting spells, making prophecies, puns and witticisms, et cetera. All that sort of conjuring with words was increasingly dismissed by the new, rational society of the eighteenth century as silly, or indeed, as they significantly called it, childish. The mad were thus reduced to children, people who were pre- or sub-rational. At the same time, in the religious domain, there was a new creed in the eighteenth century of rational religion: John Locke, the philosopher, wrote a book called *The Reasonableness of Christianity*. That creed also psycho-pathologised the old transcendental flights of faith as being mere 'enthusiasm', the great slur-

word of the eighteenth century, or a form of religious melancholy, neces-
sarily devoid of any authentic divine revelation, because it was not derived
from above, as traditionally claimed, but was a kind of disease of the guts.
It came from biliousness of the bowels: that is where the Methodists, the
Quakers and others got their religious transports from, not from the divine
Logos. One eighteenth-century physician, Nicholas Robinson, who was a
great follower, significantly, of the physics of Sir Isaac Newton, said of the
Quakers that they were subject to strong convulsive fits, and that their
spoutings were nothing but the stronger impulses of a warm brain:

> When the brain is once well warm'd, then every groundless Opinion ...
> is an Illumination from the Spirit of God, and of divine Authority, and
> every Impulse that drives them on to any odd and ridiculous Action, is
> immediately a divine call from Heaven ....[15]

Religious sectories might claim that God used his prophets as mouthpieces
for his word, a bit like the experience of John Perceval referred to earlier,
but increasingly they were referred to as, in that classic phrase, the religious
'lunatic fringe'. Voices from beyond had become too disturbing and sub-
versive, and psychological medicine adopted a regulatory role in distinguishing between, as it were, proper, moderate, common sense, polite
religion, and, on the other hand, the religion that was fit for 'the bin'. It
was noted in the eighteenth century just how many Methodists, for
example, were put inside, because their religion was too emotional and was
thought therefore to be disturbed because it was disturbing. In the same
way, in the nineteenth century lots of argumentative women got stigmatised, and some got certified, and some got put away, because their claim
for political rights, or for higher education, was always said to be hysterical.
Psychiatric terms are very good put-downs of people whose politics and
aspirations one wishes to squash.

Rationalism and scientific medicine thus silenced, or at least rendered
meaningless, what it didn't want to hear. There was also a long tradition
of eliding mental disturbance with speech disturbance. Think in our language of the double meaning of the word 'dumb': mute, but also, stupid.
Melancholics had traditionally been identified by their moody brooding,
maniacs by their animalistic roarings, and the so-called lycanthropes by
their alleged baying at the moon. And as psychiatric classifications came to
be elaborated in the nineteenth century, then quirks and impairments
of speech came to be definitive of particular psychiatric diagnostic syndromes. Aphasia became defined as a typical defect of speech; logorrhoea,
the incapacity to stop speaking; coprolalia, speaking dirty; et cetera.[16]
Incommunicative autism became one of the diagnostic signs for the
emergent concept of schizophrenia in the early twentieth century. And
of course one wonders how many patients who authentically suffered

neurological defects which deranged their speech were called mad or insane, although all they had were neurological disorders.

Intellectual trends in emergent psychiatry imposed a kind of sound barrier between doctors and patients. The sick, it was often said, needed quiet, calm, freedom from interference, and that meant silence. From the 1770s one of the pioneering private madhouse keepers in England, a man called William Perfect, detained patients in solitary confinement in silence for months on end, in the belief that this was therapeutically optimal, or, as he might have said, 'perfect'. Of one especially confused patient, who had his head racked with financial anxieties – and this again may be a topical reference – Perfect says, 'I never suffered him to be spoken with'. The outcome of that? He made a complete recovery, until finally he was able to communicate 'rationally and just'.[17] And similar strategies – bans on company, on correspondence, and all the other supposedly counter-productive stimuli – characterise the famous or notorious rest cure for that new condition, emergent in the late nineteenth century, of neurasthenia. Neurasthenics – often hysterical women – were put into special institutions. They were kept silent; they were told not to speak; they were not allowed to write; and they were fed up on vast quantities of milk, butter, dairy products, rice puddings, et cetera, in order to fatten them up, and to make them, if you like, bovine. You could almost imagine them mooing at the end of it all. That was the treatment that Virgina Woolf experienced when she had a breakdown, and it was also characteristic of the experience of the American writer, Charlotte Perkins Gilman, who wrote that wonderful novella, *The Yellow Wallpaper*.

My point is that this muting of the mad was not simply an abuse imposed by ignorant, cruel and benighted asylum keepers, but was actually seen as a prize feature of enlightened and progressive and apparently successful therapies. At the distinguished York retreat, set up around 1800 and the beacon of enlightened institutions in England throughout the Victorian period, it was positively policy to refuse to enter into discussion with any patients about their delusions. Samuel Tuke, the grandson of William Tuke, the founder of the York retreat, wrote:

> In regard to melancholics, conversation on the subject of their despondency is found to be highly injudicious. The very opposite method is pursued. Every means is taken to seduce the mind from its favourite but unhappy musings, by bodily exercise, walks, conversation, reading, and other innocent recreations.[18]

This strategy was widely endorsed. After all, if madness was, as people said, a form of deluded imagination, then it was folly indeed to dwell upon it. And it had, above all, no meaning. Nothing that mad people said would actually give you insight into what was wrong with them, and therefore it was better not to hear it, to take it too seriously, or to encourage it. There is an astonishing book by the physician to Bedlam (Bethlem) asylum in London, John Haslam, called *The Illustrations of Madness*, published in 1810, which records the delusions of one particular patient, a man called James Tilley Matthews. He claimed to be suffering from persecution by a Mesmerically operated machine, a sort of hypnosis machine, which bombarded him with such tortures as:

> *'lobster-cracking', 'stomach-skinning', 'apoplexy-working with the nutmeg grater', 'foot-curving, lethargy-making, spark-exploding, knee-nailing, burning-out, eye-screwing, sight-stopping, roof-stringing, vital-tearing, and fibre-ripping'.*[19]

Haslam, the doctor, records all this – to what end? All he wishes to prove is that this man was mad, but he stops short there. He is not interested in what it might actually tell us about what's wrong with Matthews, or about how best then to overcome these conditions.

So far I have suggested that there was a kind of movement, an active movement, in much early psychiatry – to some extent associated with the asylum movement, with locking people up, – which took the view that the voice of the mad was meaningless, and ought not to be listened to. Ironically this also proved to be the case, in some respects, with the talking cure itself in the twentieth century, with Freudian psychoanalysis. Freudian psychoanalysis classically is, or is meant to be, the therapy that does listen to patients. That is how you get to Hunter and Macalpine's claim that psychoanalysis, psychiatry in the twentieth century had taken a wrong turning, Freudianism was a mistake in promoting listening. But was it really like that? If you look at what Freud recommended as the proper analytic technique, it is not a dialogue between the therapist and the patient at all. The therapist sits there silently behind the patient, occasionally saying 'ah ha', and nudging the patient along, and the patient does all the talking. The analyst is not, as it were, meant to operate on the wavelength of what the patient is saying, but is all the time meant to be decoding what the patient is saying, or listening to what the patient is not saying, hearing the unconscious, working out the hidden meanings (hidden from the patient) of the consciousness itself. I think Hunter and Macalpine were mistaken in believing that Freudianism was a new aberration. There was nothing new about psychiatry not actually listening to the mad, but only looking at them or silencing them.

As I have said, I am not a psychiatrist, I am a historian. How does a historian approach the history of madness? How does the historian get under the skin of what has been going on in the encounters between doctors and psychiatric patients over the centuries? There are many ways to write the history of psychiatry: it can be written in a long-term chronological narrative of the state of the psychiatric profession, of the law, of funding anxieties, of psycho-pharmaceuticals, and so on. These are all essential aspects of the history of psychiatry. But another key aspect, because this is where it all stems from, is the minds of disturbed people themselves, and the way in which there have been these encounters between the disturbed and the doctors. One of the very remarkable developments of history itself over the last twenty or thirty years is that the doing of History has got away from grand narratives, huge teleological histories from the beginning to the end, for example, in the Marxist way of seeing everything as being determined by class, or by economics, or by politics. What we get increasingly is what social historians call 'micro-histories', the histories of small-scale encounters at the workplace, within the family, histories of private life, histories of popular culture, histories of life-styles, histories of what used to be called the trivial, but nowadays are seen to be the politics of everyday life – the politics of the body, the politics of gender. Historians are now fascinated by this micro-historical approach, and it has been very, very revealing indeed.

Can we do that sort of micro-politics for psychiatry? Can we actually see what went on in the minds of mad people despite the fact that they were largely silenced? Couldn't a critic, an objector say, 'well, where can we get any evidence as to what mad people thought, experienced, suffered, said? How would you know?' What has come to light, largely from new archival studies, are the rich records of aspects of doctor-patient encounters in the past, and records, often written down by doctors, of what mad people were actually, allegedly, saying. There is an astonishing book called *Mystical Bedlam*, written by an American historian, Michael MacDonald, which records a seventeenth-century clergyman of the Church of England who doubled as a mad doctor, a man called Richard Napier, a contemporary and friend of Robert Burton, who wrote the great *Anatomy of Melancholy*.[20] Richard Napier recorded thousands of case studies of mad people he treated and by a lucky chance his case histories have actually survived. Because I think he was an accurate and honest recorder of what the patients said to him, we now know, by a miracle, the miseries, the complaints, the fears, the anxieties, the phobias, the paranoias of two thousand mad people from the early part of the seventeenth century. Now, it could be that there is a built-in distortion here because it is all mediated through the doctor and somehow we don't get it from the horse's mouth. Other sorts of evidence are obviously tainted. The classic mad person you get in Shakespeare's plays, or in Gothic novels, or in sentimental novels, is obviously a literary construction: whether or not there's any truth in this type, or whether it is only a matter of sentimental projection or dramatic licence is hard to say. But it is a matter of fact that there are hundreds of published and unpublished autobiographical writings by mad people: I mentioned John Perceval's earlier. Of course they are unreliable, they are bound to be. Here were exceptional people, often writing in protest about being incarcerated by society, or writing to vindicate themselves against people who didn't understand them, and therefore there is often something very peculiar yet revealing in what they write. One of my favourite autobiographies, unpublished, in the British Library, about a million and a half words, is from the end of the seventeenth century, by a Member of Parliament called Goodwin Wharton.[21] He explains in his diary that he impregnated his mistress 106 times, at the very same time as he was having affairs with three successive queens of England. Now clearly this can't just be taken as fact: a historian needs to read between the lines and imaginatively reconstruct some of this, and to think what is actually going on when there is a member of the cabinet who is having these sorts of fantasies and delusions. Sometimes we are lucky in having two sides of the case: what a mad person thought, and then what an institution thought, or a doctor thought. There is an interesting pamphlet by a man called Urbane Metcalfe, who was an inmate of Bethlem asylum in London, and who thought that he was heir to the throne of Denmark, rather like Hamlet.[22] He denounces Bethlem hospital as brutal, brutalising, and corrupt. The asylum records record him as a trouble-maker. Now, doubtless both of those were true, and the historian has to integrate both sides of the story, but that's what historians are having to do with evidence all the time.

I want, just before I draw this talk to a conclusion, to give three very brief examples of where we possess fascinating and detailed testimony by mad people from the past, which then gives food for thought for the historian to try and reconstruct the history of madness.

One of them was a patient of Freud, the Russian known as Sergius P., who was, as many of you will know, Freud's 'Wolf-Man'. In Freud's case history, he analyses the Wolf-Man's dream of white wolves with bushy tails, and he decodes the white wolves with bushy tails into a story about how the young Wolf-Man saw his parents copulating.[23] And then there is a second story about the Wolf-Man, written in 1928 by the second person who analysed him, a patient and student of Freud called Ruth Mack Brunswick [and a third, by the psycho-analyst Muriel Gardiner, who had been analysed by Brunswick and who assisted the Wolf-Man in fleeing to the United States just before the Second World War].[24] And then, interestingly, in the 1960s, the Wolf-Man, who by then was in his eighties, was interviewed by a journalist, Karin Obholzer. Obholzer asks what the Wolf-Man made of Freud's analysis of his dreams.' And he says – very aristocratically – 'I never thought much of dream interpretation, you know... . It's all terribly far-fetched'. She asks further what he made

of Freud's deduction that he was only sexually functional if he could
have sex 'from behind':

W: 'Well, that was never absolute, you know ....'

'... that also depends on the woman, how she is built.'

'With Therese [his wife], if you insist on details, the first coitus was that
she sat on top of me.'

O: 'That would be the precise opposite....'

W: 'I ask myself the following: Are we sitting in judgement on psychoanalysis? (*laughs*)[25]

Obholzer questions him about whether Freud was dispassionate, and the
Wolf-Man answers:

'Freud was a genius even though not everything he said was true.'

'When he had explained everything to me, I said to him, "All right
then, I agree, but I am going to check whether it is correct." And he said:
"Don't start that. Because the moment you try to view things critically,
your treatment will get nowhere. I will help you, whether you now believe
in it, or not." So I naturally gave up the idea of any further criticism.'[26]

So there are at least four takes on the Wolf-Man. There's Freud's Wolf-Man;
there's Ruth Mack Brunswick's Wolf-Man; there's Muriel Gardiner's Wolf-
Man; and there's the Wolf-Man's Wolf-Man, at various stages in his life.
Now, none of them is simply the truth, but if we have several bits of
evidence it helps quite a lot.

Now I want to go back to James Tilley Matthews, the man who had all
the delusions about his persecution by the Mesmeric machine, because we
have John Haslam's record of all this, but we also have many manuscript
writings in James Tilley Matthews's own hand, which were preserved by
Bethlem, and these show very clearly that Matthews thought he was being
persecuted by the machines. [Matthews was a London tea-merchant who
had been attracted by French revolutionary ideas and by the popular philosophy of Mesmerism (a hypnotic technique of mind control through eyes,
voice or 'rays', developed by the Viennese physician Franz Anton Mesmer).
Matthews hoped to promote peace between France and England, with the
help of Lord Liverpool, and following Mesmeric philosophy; when the
Jacobins seized power, however, he became suspect both for his politics
and his interest in Mesmerism, and was imprisoned in France. When he

returned to Britain in 1796, he was persuaded that he had sole knowledge of a French revolutionary plot to gain all state secrets and military control, in order to republicanise Britain and Ireland. The plot would use Mesmeric machines, in particular 'airlooms', which would transmit rays: Matthews saw his own tortures as effected by the conspirators in this way. He wrote repeated letters warning of the plot to the government, and in particular, to Lord Liverpool. Ignored, he came to believe in Liverpool's treachery, and that of the government more generally: he accused them to the House of Commons, and was examined by the Privy Council before being committed to Bethlem. For him, of course, this was proof of the conspiracy against him.] At the same time that he suffered the persecutions of machines, he obviously was being persecuted in a different way by the government. [Not only his family, but also their lawyers and physicians, including the respected doctors Birkbeck and Clutterbuck, attempted to secure his release, but to no avail. From the minutes of committee meetings in Bethlem, it is clear that political pressure was exerted on the Governors not to free Matthews: Lord Liverpool and Lord Sidmouth intervened directly in 1809, 1813 and 1814. Unsurprisingly, the Governors of Bethlem] refused to let Matthews out even though some of the leading doctors in the country said that he was sane. So his feelings of persecution were an accurate record, if you like, of being persecuted.[27]

Lastly, I'd just like to mention a third interesting case, the memoirs of Daniel Schreber, a German judge, and another person whom Freud analysed, though at a distance. [Freud interpreted Schreber's paranoia as caused by repressed homosexual desire for his psychiatrist, which sublimated his desire for his dead father and brother.][28] Schreber's [own view of things was rather different, though his memoirs are deeply concerned with his sexual identity'[29]: he saw his first breakdown in 1884 as the result of overwork; his second, in 1894, was marked first by depression and then a belief that he was assailed by 'nervous disease'. Schreber associated the nerves with the soul and with God, believing that men could gain mastery through control of the nerves of others, a theory similar to that of Matthews regarding Mesmeric control. Schreber believed that at God's command his doctor, Flechsig, was plotting the murder of his soul; Flechsig would also gain his body, changed into female form. His memoirs detail his psychosis: his growing sense of being bodily and mentally invaded, and becoming 'unmanned'. Gradually, he came to believe that he was the last surviving human, and that he would be the instrument for the renewal of the human race though divine conception, a second Virgin Birth. His ideas, however bizarre, are placed in the context of Christian eschatology and apocalyptic science, while he interprets the medical ideas of his day as symptomatic of the degeneracy of civilisation. Schreber's memoirs thus engage with the powerful and dangerous notions of his time, of racial degeneration and purification.] They are full of anti-Semitism, and of anti-Slav sentiment, they glorify the Aryan race, and reading them is almost like reading a pre-echo of *Mein Kampf* when it comes to racial ideas. And this is in a sense what I want to suggest: that there is a meaning in madness: there are ideas, models, fantasies shared by mad people and by society at large. The fantasies, the paranoias of mad people are not unique to themselves. They draw upon information, ideas, influences that come from society at large, and then re-work them.

Let me offer a concluding remark or two. The anthropologist Mary Douglas said that dirt is matter out of place. You could say that madness has become sound out of place, or words out of place, since the seventeenth century. Increasingly what you could call inappropriate vocalisations became part of the definition of psychopathology. If you go back to an earlier world, a rural world, an oral world, a peasant world, there are all sorts of sounds all over the place, and they are taken for granted. It's assumed that God speaks to humans. It's assumed that there is a music of the spheres. It's assumed that demons talk to you. It's assumed that a serpent in the Garden of Eden spoke to Adam and Eve. There is all sorts of speaking, and it's not automatically seen as being mad. Saint Francis talked to the animals. Apollo sang to them. All of that now seems deeply strange to us. We have changed our cultural orientation in the era of the cell-phone and the walkman. These are our ways in which noises come to us in a disembodied way, legitimately. We have not yet, unfortunately, got to the stage where people using cell-phones endlessly are thought to be suffering from some disorder! It is all relative, in other words. Madness changes its definition according to the culture in which it works, and what I've been suggesting here is that one of the prime axes upon which the understanding of madness and sanity has changed and moved over the last few centuries is the question of the meaningfulness of appropriate speech. And for that very reason we have in the historical record abundant documentation of appropriate and inappropriate speech, which is what allows the history of madness to be written.

Notes

1 Richard Hunter and Ida Macalpine, *George III and the Mad-Business* (London, 1969).
2 Richard Hunter and Ida Macalpine, *Psychiatry for the Poor. 1851 Colney Hatch Asylum: Friern Hospital 1973. A Medical and Social History*, Psychiatric Monographs Series 9 (London, 1974), pp. 183–84. See also Roy Porter, *Madness: A Brief History* (Oxford, 2002) pp. 156–57.
3 See Hunter and Macalpine, *Psychiatry for the Poor*, p. 196.
4 John Thomas Perceval, *Perceval's Narrative: A Patient's Account of his Psychosis, 1830–1832*, ed. Gregory Bateson (London, 1962), pp. 18, 46. For the full version of Perceval's account, see *A Narrative of the Treatment Received by a Gentleman, During a State of Mental Derangement ...*, 2 vols (London, 1838, 1840). For a more extended discussion of Perceval's narrative, see Roy Porter, *A Social History of*

Madness: Stories of the Insane (London, 1987, 1996), pp. 167–88 (see esp. pp. 182, 185). See also Andrew Scull, *The Most Solitary of Afflictions: Madness and Society in Britain 1700–1900* (New Haven, 1993) p. 80.

5 Perceval, p. 29.
6 Perceval, p. 95.
7 Perceval, p. 120.
8 Perceval, p. 119.
9 Perceval, p. 121.
10 Donald McI. Johnson and Norman Dodds, eds, *The Plea for the Silent* (London, 1957), p. 51. See also Porter, *Madness*, p. 160.
11 Nicholas Culpeper, *Culpeper's 'School of Physick'*, *or the Experimental Practice of the Whole Art* (London, 1659), 'Of Madness', p. 353, also cited by Michael MacDonald, *Mystical Bedlam: Madness, Anxiety and Healing in Seventeenth-Century England*, Cambridge Monographs in the History of Medicine (Cambridge, 1981) p. 139.
12 Michel Foucault, *Madness and Civilization: A History of Insanity in the Age of Reason*, trans. Richard Howard (London, 1967, 1989) p. 78. Originally published as *Folie et déraison: histoire de la folie à l'âge classique*, Civilisations d'hier et d'aujourd'hui (Paris, 1961).
13 See also Porter, *Madness*, p. 158.
14 Alexander Pope, *Essay on Criticism*, in *The Poems of Alexander Pope*, ed. John Butt, 2nd edn (London, 1965), Part II, line 365.
15 Nicholas Robinson, *A New System of the Spleen* ... (London, 1729) p. 247. See also Porter, *Madness*, pp. 30, 126.
16 See also Hunter and Macalpine, *Psychiatry for the Poor*, pp. 206–207.
17 William Perfect, *Select Cases in the Different Species of Insanity, Lunacy, or Madness...* (Rochester, 1787) pp. 4, 6.
18 Samuel Tuke, *Description of the Retreat: An Institution Near York for Insane Persons of the Society of Friends* (York, 1815) pp. 151–52. A facsimile edition is introduced by Richard Hunter and Ida Macalpine (London, 1964). This passage is also cited by Andrew Scull, Charlotte Mackenzie and Nicolas Hervey, *Masters of Bedlam: The Transformation of the Mad-Doctoring Trade* (Princeton, 1996) pp. 101–102, note 187.
19 John Haslam, *Illustrations of Madness* ... (London, 1810) pp. 32–38. See also the Tavistock reprint edition, introduced by Roy Porter (London, 1989) and Porter, *A Social History*, p. 56, Scull, *The Most Striking of Afflictions*, p. 95, note 154, and Patricia Allderidge, 'Bedlam: fact or fantasy', in W. F. Bynum, Roy Porter and Michael Shepherd, *The Anatomy of Madness: Essays in the History of Psychiatry*, 3 vols (London, 1985) vol. 2: *Institutions and Society*, pp. 17–33 (p. 34 and notes 111–112).
20 See above, note 6.
21 See Porter, *Social History*, p. 30.
22 Urbane Metcalfe, *The Interior of Bethlehem Hospital, Humbly Addressed to His Royal Highness the Duke of Sussex and the Other Governors* (London, 1818). See also Porter, *Madness*, p. 161.
23 Sigmund Freud, *From the History of an Infantile Neurosis* (1918 [1914]), in *The Standard Edition of the Complete Psychological Works of Sigmund Freud*, ed. and trans. James Strachey et al., 24 vols (London, 1953–74) vol. 17, pp. 1–122. For a fuller discussion, see Porter, *Social History*, pp. 223–28.
24 For both accounts, printed together with the Wolf-Man's memoirs and his re-collections of Freud, see Muriel Gardiner, ed., *The Wolf-Man and Sigmund Freud*, The International Psycho-Analytical Library 88 (London, 1972).

25 Karin Obholzer, *The Wolf-Man Sixty Years Later: Conversations with Freud's Controversial Patient,* trans. Michael Shaw (London, 1982 (originally published in German, 1980)) pp. 35, 133–34.

26 Obholzer, pp. 30–31.

27 For a full discussion of the case, from which this description is largely drawn, see Porter, *Social History,* pp. 54–59, Scull, *The Most Striking of Afflictions,* p. 95, note 154, and Scull, MacKenzie and Hervey, *Masters of Bedlam,* p. 34 and, for discussion of the Bethlem records, notes 111–12.

28 See Freud, 'Psycho-analytic Notes on an Autobiographical Account of a Case of Paranoia (Dementia Paranoides)', *Standard Edition,* vol. 12, pp. 3–84.

29 This explanatory passage is largely based on Porter's full discussion in *Social History,* pp. 146–66. For Schreber's memoirs, see Daniel Paul Schreber, *Memoirs of my Nervous Illness,* trans. and ed. Ida Macalpine and Richard A. Hunter (London: Dawson, 1955).

2
Doctors as Performance Artists

Michael O'Donnell

One drowsy summer afternoon, as I endured a lecture on 'Communication Pathways in the Doctor-Patient Relationship' – I really should have known better – I was granted a flash of hindsight. It would sound more impressive if I called it insight but for some of us, insight is often a resolution of reflections on the past.

For some fifty years, as a voyeur of medicine, I had tried to analyse the qualities possessed by doctors whom patients feel better for seeing, regardless of the treatment they prescribe – doctors whom some call 'healers'. That afternoon, as the lecturer – who had introduced himself, without a blush, as 'a communications expert' – droned along his own well-trodden pathway, the reaction of his audience revealed the true nature of his expertise. He was an accomplished bore.

At first I was amused. Then, as he persisted in his selfishness and my amusement turned to anger, there came my moment of Damascene road rage. Suddenly I grasped an idea that had been marinating in my brain for half a century. I recognised that the 'healing' relationship that intrigued me was akin to that which exists between performer and audience, and that doctors could learn much about their craft from the work of actors, dramatists, and novelists.

This collection of essays deals with the links, sometimes uneasy, between medicine, madness, and literature. In the first half of my working life, when I earned my living as a doctor, I was conditioned to define true 'madness' as an assortment of well-defined diseases of the mind and less well-defined eccentricities, insecurities, and perceived inadequacies that people brought to my surgery in the same way they brought their inflamed appendices, their sinister tumours, their crumbling joints, their sore throats and their haemorrhoids. Occasionally I would affect a 'cure'; sometimes I could modify their symptoms. Yet whatever their 'madness' or 'unwellness', the real challenge was to help them achieve some sort of harmony with their environment.

In pursuit of this extravagant ambition I discovered that some of the most helpful textbooks could be found on library shelves labelled

'Literature'. Not every shelf, mark you. When later I use the word 'literature' I will use it to describe writing that endures because people enjoy reading and re-reading it, watching it, or listening to it being performed – a definition influenced by Terry Eagleton's observation:

> The reason why the vast majority of people read poems, novels and plays is because they find them pleasurable. This fact is so obvious that it is hardly ever mentioned in universities. It is, admittedly, difficult to spend some years studying literature in most universities and still find it pleasurable at the end: many university literature courses seem to be constructed to prevent this from happening, and those who emerge still able to enjoy literary works might be considered either heroic or perverse.[1]

I started my career as a medical voyeur at an early age. My father was a GP in a Yorkshire village that for the first decade of the twentieth century was a huddle of cottages and farmhouses on the side of a hill. Then in 1912 a mining company sank a shaft in the valley below, created Yorkshire Main Colliery, and surrounded it with a warren of back to back terraces to house the miners it imported to extract the coal. In the 1930s most of my father's patients were miners and their families, some were farmers and farm labourers, and a few were the managers and engineers who served the needs of the pit and the teachers and shopkeepers who served the needs of the village.

Early in my childhood my father used to take me with him in his car, and sometimes into a house, when he indulged in that strange habit that doctors once had of visiting the sick. Up to the age of ten or eleven I was even allowed during school holidays to sit in a corner of his consulting room until despatched to the treatment room whenever he or his patient sought privacy.

In the first half of the twentieth century, that wasn't an unusual practice. Nor confined to these islands. Ten years before, Lewis Thomas, the American medical scientist and essayist, had sat beside his GP father in his car while he did his rounds on Long Island. His father like mine enjoyed his son's company, and the young Lewis Thomas, like the young me, enjoyed listening to his father and discovering what he got up to when he was out of the house. 'Watching my father's work,' wrote Thomas, 'was the most everyday part of my childhood'.[2]

As I watched my father work I discovered that, outside our home, he became a performer who, when treating patients, would suit his performance to the occasion. Most often he would play the kindly, wise, and sympathetic counsellor, sometimes he would be the cheery motivator driving away dull care, and I once saw him, when dealing with a husband who had punched his wife in the face, give a terrifyingly convincing performance of an avenging devil.

But then every performance was convincing and later, when I worked as his assistant for a couple of weeks while his colleague was on holiday, I realised that he had acquired much of his understanding of medicine from his patients, in the way that performers learn from their audience. True, he picked up useful knowledge from books and journals but he screened everything he read through the filter of his own experience.

I've since met many doctors who performed in much the same way and I now recognise that the empathy they had with their patients, the ability to see the world exactly as it appeared in the eyes of their audience, was one of the elusive qualities that create a good 'healer', a doctor whom patients feel better for seeing. I've also recognised that the source of this ability to think oneself into the minds of others is much the same for effective doctors as it is for effective actors and effective writers.

For nearly every human action, I suggest, you can define two reasons: the good reason and the real reason. And performers, be they actors, writers, or doctors, share an interest in defining the real reason. Doctors who are 'good healers' establish contact with the person who lurks behind the social façade. The Swedish actor and novelist Henning Mankell speaks for both his crafts when he describes how performance involves, 'Reading between the lines, looking for the subtext.'[3]

Performing and role playing

There is a crucial distinction between performing, which is a creative activity, and the playing of roles, which is not. Performers need an audience and are influenced by it; role-players are concerned only with satisfying themselves.

The medical performer is more a jazz musician for whom every performance is something new than a pop musician twanging out the same track over and over again; a concert pianist responding to an audience rather than a pianola player – who come to think of it is a literal roll player.

Unlike role-playing, performance demands emotional engagement from both performer and audience. When a performer gets it right, the audience responds and plays its part and good performers fuel that audience reaction by modifying their own behaviour. Richard Eyre, a former director of the National Theatre, once said, 'Great performances are written in water'. And that is both their strength and their sadness.

Successful performances reward not just the audience but the performer. Indeed, the greatest reward to come a performer's way is the audience response: the magical moment when an actor discovers that a line delivered in a certain way can set off an eruption of laughter or provoke silence, or tears, or a growl of anger; the moment when a doctor sees the dawn of self-confidence in a patient, or a teacher sees the dawn of understanding in a student.

In medicine, as in the theatre or the classroom, performers will evoke this response only if they are constantly aware of audience reaction. To describe how I learned that lesson I need to call on my father once again, because he was the first person to teach it to me. I later had to re-learn it many times but in life, as in love, the first time is usually the most memorable ... if not necessarily the most enjoyable.

The case of the worried miner

A year or so after I qualified as a doctor, and while I was doing that holiday locum in my father's practice, I was called one day to see a miner who'd taken to his bed with vague abdominal symptoms. I can see him now: thin-face, high-forehead, watching anxiously while I examined and re-examined him, did lots of investigations, yet detected nothing abnormal. I was so worried about him that I took to visiting him every day and watched him daily grow more ill. Because I was insensitive to audience reaction I couldn't see that the more I worried about him, the more he worried about himself.

In desperation I called in my father for a second opinion and, again, I can see him bursting into the patient's bedroom radiating good cheer. 'Now George, what the hell have you being doing to my son?' he said. 'You should be ashamed of yourself, worrying him out of his wits.' He then sat on the side of the bed engaging in cheery conversation with my patient who, for the first time since I'd seen him, allowed that drawn face to melt into a smile. My father then examined him as thoroughly as I had, chatting away merrily as he did so, and extracting the news that George was having problems with his foreman who seemed to have it in for him.

When he'd finished his examination, my father prescribed the treatment. 'You'd best get out of bed,' he said. 'Lying there is doing you no good. I think you've let this business at the pit get to your stomach but you need to be up and about. I'll give you a note to Ernie Bicknell to help you get on a different shift. In the meantime don't start putting the fear of God into well-meaning young doctors.'

As we left the room I turned and saw that the thin worried face that I'd visited daily had fattened into a broad expansive grin. The anxiety that had devoured him – and which those who worked alongside him in the pit or drank alongside him in the pub might have called madness, or more likely 'daftness' – had vanished in the twinkling of my father's eye.

Truth and consequences

Awareness of audience response is one essential ingredient of performance. There is another. In medicine, as in the theatre, the quality that distinguishes performing from role-playing is that it be truthful – even if the truth exists only in the eyes and ears of the audience. The audience perceives a real person, real emotion; the skill of the performer blinds them to the artifice that has to be employed.

The late Sir Alec Guinness once described the process to me over the relics of a memorable lunch. All of the body and ninety-nine hundredths of the mind, he said, must be devoted to producing a convincing truthful performance. Yet in a tiny corner – that remaining hundredth of the mind – sits the pilot with his hands on the controls, coolly monitoring the timing, the audience reaction, remembering the lines, the rehearsed moves, intonations, pauses, while knowing that a false move on his part will shatter the illusion of a seemingly impromptu physical performance.

Getting that creative balance right makes the difference between a theatrical performance that is magical and one that is mechanical and mundane. Getting the balance right in a medical consultation makes the difference between one that is therapeutic and one that is mechanical and mundane.

In medicine as in the theatre, allowing the artifice to show can have catastrophic effects. In the early days of the Samaritans, when I was involved in training volunteers, I soon learned how people under stress get greater reassurance from fellow human beings who may themselves may be anxious, uncertain, and unauthoritative but show genuine concern, than they get from those who are so occupied turning over textbook pages in their minds that they radiate not one glow of the humanity that they share with their client.

That experience taught me that the way to help people develop a healing presence is to nurture their individual gifts rather than try to impose a false persona upon them. It also taught me never to try as doctor to reassure, advise, or seek to win trust by assuming a false persona. It's a lesson that actors learn early in their training. As the Principal of a drama school put it:

> An actor working at full pitch operates with the substance of his or her own life.... The degree to which a performance is convincing often reflects the extent to which the actor is able to draw truthfully on his or her own essence.[4]

Even the most versatile actors know there is a limit to the range of parts they can play, imposed by their personality, their physical shape and what that accomplished actress and teacher Athene Seyler called their 'spiritual comprehension' of the role they want to play:

> There is one actor I know well who can suggest cruelty, tenderness, weakness, strength, stupidity and intelligence: but his one failure is in expressing coarseness. He may assume the externals of a coarse-minded

man in his make-up, way of walking, clothes and manner, but his approach to the character is imposed from outside and he never succeeds in convincing the audience of its truth.[5]

These limitations on performance are not confined to the theatre. Alec Guinness's commonplace book records a remark by Samuel Johnson: 'Almost all absurdity of conduct arises from the imitation of those we cannot resemble'.[6]

There are, of course, doctors so lucky in their genes that their personae need no nurturing. In a stage direction in *The Doctor's Dilemma*, Bernard Shaw describes the bombastic Sir Ralph Bloomfield Bonnington:

> He radiates an enormous self-confidence, cheering, reassuring, healing by the mere incompatibility of disease or anxiety with his welcome presence. Even broken bones, it is said, have been known to unite at the sound of his voice.[7]

That sort of self confidence can be highly reassuring to patients, even those of some intelligence. Indeed it is commonly found in doctors who specialise in diseases of the rich. At first glance it may look like role-playing but the skill with which the power of the personality is switched to high or low or to some point in between defines it as a true performance.

This also shows that a therapeutic relationship between performer and audience does not have to be a sympathetic one. What makes the performance therapeutic is that it creates an emotional link. When I was in general practice I read a report of research suggesting that the most effective way of getting rid of warts was not to cut them off or to freeze them but to 'charm' them. I was not surprised. I had seen a surgeon in our local hospital achieve a high cure rate in children by making mystic signs over the wart while muttering Jabberwocky phrases in a broad Devonian accent.

Such power is rarely bestowed by the sort of role-playing favoured by doctors who pride themselves on their 'bedside manner', by which they too often mean charm or sympathy 'switched on' as a deliberate technique rather than generated by emotion: the smile swiftly wiped on and even more swiftly wiped off, the show of interest that lives only in the lips and cheeks while the eyes remain dead. These tricks convey the sincerity of a television game-show host, rarely reassure patients, and endow their perpetrators with the charm of a party political broadcast.

Cartoon doctors

One of the pernicious effects of repetitive role-playing is that it leads inevitably to caricature. I once saw an exhibition of photographs and cartoons of Richard Nixon that demonstrated how the longer he hung on to the American presidency the more he grew to resemble the newspaper caricatures. Caricature is dangerous because role players all too easily become role models. Impressionable students start to model themselves on 'characters' they feel they should admire. Even more dangerously, as those students grow older, they come to regard themselves as the embodiment of those they once admired.

This natural progress from admiration to imitation is not confined to medicine. In his history of Shakespearean biography, Samuel Schoenbaum shows how all of Shakespeare's biographers tend to portray the great man as someone remarkably like themselves. This common human failing has helped perpetuate some of the most dangerous stereotypes in medicine.

- The decisive surgeon who is sometimes mistaken but never in doubt
- The reactionary grouch who prides himself on being 'one of the old school' which, as Dickens points out in *Bleak House*, is any school that seems never to have been young
- The medical chauvinists whose exploits are recorded by colleagues like Dr Luisa Dillner:

> When considering the attitude of male obstetricians and gynaecologists, you have to remember they are predominantly surgeons. This makes them automatically autocratic. Many genuinely have difficulty with the concept that's what's yours isn't necessarily theirs to remove.[8]

and by Dr Phil Hammond who, when lecturing in Birmingham in 1995, heard a student describe what happened when she assisted a surgeon:

> First he asked me if I was from the Home Counties. When I said yes, he started calling me Tinkerbelle and said I looked the sort of girl who'd had a horse between my legs. Then he asked me if I'd lost my virginity up against the wall of a horse-box while my mother was outside watching a gymkhana. The registrar and the other theatre staff started laughing too. It was like being in a monkey house. At the end, he asked me if I minded him being sexist in theatre? 'Women like to know what men want'. Then he made a hole in the gall-bladder and said, 'Look what you've made me do.'[9]

One reason these stereotypes persist is that role-players never cast a critical eye at their own performance. They have an image of what a doctor should be and set out to play that role, assuming that if they go through the motions they will produce a convincing performance. Erving Goffman described the phenomenon: 'Many of these efforts remind one of the experiments that children perform with chemistry sets: "Follow instructions and you can be a real chemist just like the picture on the box."'[10] But then role-playing by its nature demands that the player be concerned with the picture on the box, particularly in an age when an ephemeral quality called 'image' is highly prized by those more concerned with shadow than with substance.

Whenever I write about medicine, or talk about it on radio or television, I receive invitations to contribute to meetings with titles like 'How to improve the profession's public image'. I usually refuse, I hope politely, because I've always regarded a 'good image' as akin to other abstractions like dignity, a sense of humour, or sex appeal. If you find yourself worrying about whether you've got them, you've probably got something to worry about. These are accolades that other people bestow on you if you're lucky and a good performer. Only role-players seek ways of awarding them to themselves.

Still, I recognise that some doctors, like some actors, need props to help them perform. If they're desperate, I suggest they stick to those recommended by Samuel Johnson: a top hat to give them authority, a paunch to give them dignity, and piles to give them an anxious expression.

The art that disguises art

When we watch successful performers in a television drama we get caught up in the lives and problems of the 'real' characters they portray. We forget that these are actors working to a script, the pilot in the corner of each brain remembering the lines, following the rehearsed moves, sensing where the camera is, blanking out the sight of the gaggle of gum-chewing technicians that confronts them. The 'reality' they create relies heavily on techniques but the techniques can never be allowed to show. That would shatter the illusion.

Similarly medical performers need to master the art that disguises art and some of the techniques they need are specific to their craft. One of the most useful lessons I learned from my teacher in general practice was how to turn young children into an audience: how when I visited their homes and entered their rooms I should ignore them and take an interest in everything else, pictures on the wall, the view from the window, until the children's curiosity led them to take an interest in me, stop crying, even stand up in their cots hoping to make the acquaintance of this unusual stranger.

Doctors can learn equally useful techniques from actors.

- They need to train themselves not just to listen to patients but to attend to the actual meaning of the words, even if they've heard them a hundred times before. Like actors in a long run they must beware of settling for a routine trot through the role. Each performance has to connect with a new audience.

- They must, like actors, be aware not just of what their voices are saying but of the messages conveyed by their bodies: the messages sent by their posture, the messages that lurk in their eyes and often contradict those that issue from their mouths.
- They must know how to use their voices, and their bodies, to underline the most significant phrases that they speak, the ones they hope will linger in the audience's memory.
- But, above all, they must learn not just to listen but to *respond*.

Response

I recently talked to an actor who'd just done a spell in a television 'soap' and had quite enjoyed it because he was surrounded by actors who knew their job and were used to working together. A bit like being back in weekly rep, he said. But there was one odd man out – an actor still in his 20s who had appeared in over two hundred episodes of soaps yet, maybe because that was his only experience, had one glaring defect. The others found him impossible to play to because they got nothing back from him. Dead eyes, said my friend. That's all you got. Dead eyes.

He got round the problem by talking over the young man's shoulder to other actors who did respond, a technique that can work in a television studio but not in a consulting room. As he spoke I remembered with shame times in my own career when I saw a patient who needed to be understood glancing desperately around the room as if seeking someone else who could provide the response that wasn't coming from me.

Limits of technique

Although these techniques are helpful they cannot, by themselves, transform us into good performers. In the clinic, as in the theatre, the performance has to integrate truthfully with the personality of the performer, its success depending on a near seamless elision of personal qualities with learned techniques.

One barrier to this successful elision is a strange entity which ambitious doctors strive to acquire in middle-age and which they call gravitas. Some of my most entertaining years as a medical voyeur were those I spent on the General Medical Council where I was able to observe that defining moment in a medical career when the Young Turk transmutes into an Old Fart.

Those aged over forty will recognise the symptoms. Men – most are men but an increasing number are women – who once were lively, witty, and intelligent companions suddenly assume a public persona quite at odds with the character that previously served them well. Where once they would have enlivened conversation, they make observations of paralysing mundanity. Drawn into public discussion, they rasp on earnestly and nod wisely as if naught but weighty thoughts were granted admission to their minds. And, on the slightest of excuses, they rise to their feet to make ponderous speeches. Most grievously of all, they refrain from using their private wit in public places for fear that amusing or penetrating remarks might prove 'politically inept'. As a result their role-playing is not just mundane but, to quote Richard Eyre again, their performances are 'head-burningly, ball-breakingly, bowel-churningly bad'.

The central lesion in this sad condition is atrophy of the sense of humour, a delicacy that can survive only if it is directed inwards as often and as assiduously as it is directed outwards. The alternative is a sad but logical progression. If you believe your eligibility for advancement will be judged by those who have long since lost their own sense of the ridiculous, clearly you must suppress the urge to exercise your own. As Sydney Smith said of his brother the bishop, 'He has risen by his gravity and I have been sunk by my levity'.

And as your sense of humour atrophies through lack of exercise so does your ability to mount a truthful performance. I'm sure it's the players' painfully assumed air of gravitas that makes medical and academic politics a repository of boring role-playing rather than exciting performance. William Somerset Maugham, doctor and writer, spoke for both his professions when he suggested, 'Make him laugh and he will think you a trivial fellow, but bore him in the right way and your reputation is assured'.[11]

Unlike the role-players, performers recognise the difference between being serious and being solemn. Some of medicine's finest performers are those who have discovered that a good way to survive in clinical practice is to adopt a bemused attitude to the mysteries of existence, loosely based on Gustav Mahler's observation that 'Humour is the only antidote to the poison of life'. And Nabokov could have been describing a wise GP when he said of Anton Chekhov: 'Things for him were funny and sad at the same time, but you would not see their sadness if you would not see their fun.'[12]

But then of all the writers who were also practising doctors Chekhov is the one who, for me, most clearly reveals how close the art of a writer is to that of a clinician. In his short stories and his plays the wise and observant doctor and the gifted writer become one. Doctors can learn not just from the tales in which he writes about physicians, hospitals, or medical encounters but from all those other stories in which his writing illuminates our understanding of human emotions, human character, human experience.

Re-reading his stories now I remember how much I learned from them when I was a young, insecure GP and feared I was the only confused inhabitant of a world that everyone else understood. I also remember how much they taught me when I was a not-so-young GP who still found life more complicated than orthodox medical texts would suggest.

Chekhovian interlude

Most GPs can offer you examples of the way that tragedy so often enters hand in hand with comedy. A GP friend of mine used to look after an odd couple – a middle-aged man and his elderly father who lived together in an isolated house and who were as dependent on one another, and as argumentative, as Steptoe and Son. One day the son called the doctor. When he arrived the son was busy in the kitchen but explained that his father had been 'a little bit quiet' all morning. When my friend went up to the father's bedroom he found that the old man was dead. He spent a minute or two trying to assemble the right words to break the news to a son who loved his father more that he loved any other creature on this earth. Yet when he went downstairs he found, as so often happens, that he lapsed into platitudes:

'I'm sorry to say,' he muttered, 'that your father has passed away.'
'Bloody hell,' said the son. 'I've just made him a big plate of stew.'

...but you would not see their sadness if you would not see their fun.

Distinguishing between illness and disease

In discussing medical performance art I've tried to define a form of creativity that is still underemphasised in the medical curriculum yet is a popular subject at GP postgraduate meetings where it appears in a variety of disguises. Why should that be in an age when doctors are rightly proud of the spectacular scientific and technological advances that their craft has made in the prevention and treatment of disease since the days that Lewis Thomas and I sat alongside our fathers in their cars?

Professor Walter Rosser offered one reason when he described how some 40 per cent of new disorders seen by GPs do not evolve into conditions that meet accepted criteria for a diagnosis.[13] Another is that, even when there is a diagnosis, GPs have to treat an illness rather than a disease. The two are not synonymous.

Diseases can be defined, their causes sought, organisms or mechanical defects identified. An illness is an individual event, the possession of one person whose physical condition and emotional state can determine the way the disease affects that individual life, can even determine the nature, severity, or pattern of symptoms that occur.

Doctors trained to diagnose and treat disease sometimes find it hard to cope with the individuality of illness. The narrow education enforced on most, though not all, medical students lays them open to the charge of Milton Mayer:

One of the things the average doctor doesn't have time to do is catch up with all the things he didn't learn in school, and one of the things he didn't learn in school is the nature of human society, its purpose, its history, and its needs. If medicine is necessarily a mystery to the average man, nearly everything else is necessarily a mystery to the average doctor.[14]

Doctors who seek to understand not just madness but the equally mysterious entity we call sanity need to explore beyond the confines of science. The Cambridge academic John Naughton, who has won as great acclaim as a television critic and essayist as he has as a scientist and engineer, explains why:

> The things that really matter to us – the secrets of the heart, of what it means to be an individual, the depths and heights of human experience – all are accessible, if at all, only through literature and the creative arts. Science has no purchase on them.[15]

Doctors who would like to treat illness as successfully as they treat disease should heed John Naughton's advice and head for shelves labelled 'Literature' where reside writers who can help them understand their patients' feelings of regret, betrayal, fear, loneliness ... indeed all the perplexing emotions that turn the same disease into a different illness in different individuals:

> One death may explain itself, but it throws no light upon another: the groping inquiry must begin anew. Preachers or scientists may generalise, but we know that no generality is possible about those whom we love; not one heaven awaits them, not even one oblivion. Aunt Juley, incapable of tragedy, slipped out of life with odd little laughs and apologies for having stopped in it so long.[16]

E. M. Forster writes not about death but about Aunt Juley. That's what novelists do. A character in a Philip Roth novel, defining his role as a writer, describes literature as 'the great particulariser' :

> Literature disturbs the organisation ... because it is not general. The intrinsic nature of the particular is to be particular, and the intrinsic nature of particularity is to fail to conform. ... Keeping the particular alive in a simplifying, generalising, world – that's where the battle is joined.[17]

It's also where the battle is joined in medicine. Modern 'evidence-based medicine', with its thirst for data and its enthusiasm for large-scale clinical trials, deals more and more with populations; yet clinicians deal with individuals. The stories of our lives are by definition anecdotal, yet medical journals spurn anecdote, preferring to publish reams of ill-digested data. Doctors who want to keep the particular alive have to turn for help to poets, novelists, and dramatists.

Luckily for doctors, writers sit there on our shelves waiting to illuminate areas of life beyond our experience, and to sharpen our appreciation of the humanity we share. And no matter the hour we consult them, we know that, unlike doctors, they will be putting on their best performance:

> In literature, time and distance mean nothing; you can meet the dead just as happily as the living, and they will take you into their confidence, tell you their jokes, give you the benefit of their opinions and experience, and ask for nothing in return but your eye on the book.[18]

The 'healing art'

The knowledge doctors acquire from observing and testing their patients enhances their knowledge of disease; the knowledge they absorb from literature enhances their understanding of illness. And the more a medical performance is based on understanding, the more likely it is to be therapeutic.

As doctors, we vaguely recognise this – we once talked about the 'healing art' – but we now have so many high tech toys to play with that we seem almost ashamed to acknowledge its existence, especially since accountants took over the world and demanded that success be measured in fiscal terms. Well defined entities like 'targets', 'outcome' and 'disease' are easier to manipulate in spreadsheets than complexities like 'illness' or 'madness'.

These fiscal measures of success are more attractive to politicians and hospital administrators than they are to doctors and nurses, who understand that the ultimate 'outcome', no matter how clever they are along the way, is a patient's death. At the start of my life as a medical voyeur I not only sat alongside my father in his car, I lived in the house he had built overlooking the village cemetery. He used to advise visiting doctors to move their homes to similar locations to provide them with a daily reminder of their ultimate achievement.

Scientific medicine has brought great rewards. It has expanded doctors' abilities to prevent disease, relieve pain, and extend people's lives. Yet most doctors still spend most of their time not in dramatic interventions but in helping people to survive the short time they spend on this planet in some sort of harmony with the world around them.

Doctors shouldn't be ashamed of the role that performance plays in their work; rather they should seek to understand why it is so effective. The main reason, I suspect, is that it is aimed at the right anatomical target – defined, as you might expect, not by a doctor but by a dramatist, Richard Brinsley Sheridan, who suggested that 'The heart, the seat of charity and compassion, is more accessible to the senses than the understanding.'[19]

Notes

1 T. Eagleton, *Literary Theory: An Introduction* (Oxford, 1983), p. 191.
2 Lewis Thomas, *The Youngest Science* (Oxford, 1984), pp. 6–14.
3 Henning Mankell, *The Fifth Woman* (London, 2001) p. 253.
4 P. Clements, 'Display of artistic integrity', *The Guardian*, 23 June, 2001, Letter.
5 Athene Seyler and Stephen Haggard, *The Craft of Comedy* (London, 1943) p. 18.
6 Alec Guinness, *A Commonplace Book* (London, 2000) p. 29.
7 Bernard Shaw, *The Doctor's Dilemma* (London, 1946) p. 104.
8 Luisa Dillner, *The Guardian*, May 14, 1998, Health page.
9 Phil Hammond and Michael Mosley, *Trust Me I'm a Doctor* (London, 1999) p. 15.
10 Erving Goffman, *Relations in Public* (London, 1971) p. xviii.
11 W. Somerset Maugham, *Gentleman in the Parlour* (London, 1930) Ch. 11.
12 Shelby Foote, ed., *Anton Chekhov: Later Short Stories 1888–1903* (New York, 1999), Introduction.
13 W. W. Rosser, 'Evidence and primary care', *Lancet* 353 (1999) pp. 661–64.
14 Milton Mayer, 'Learned medical men?', *Monitor Weekly*, 26 January, 1994, p. 56.
15 John Naughton, 'Notes on life, liberty, and the pursuit of power', *Observer*, July 9, 1995.
16 E. M. Forster, *Howard's End* (London, 1989) p. 270.
17 Philip Roth, *I Married a Communist* (London, 1999) p. 224.
18 Ruth Holland, ed., *A Sense of Asher: A New Miscellany* (London, 1983) Introduction.
19 W. Sichel, *Sheridan* (London, 1909) vol. I, p. 598.

3
Madness in Literature:
Device and Understanding

Robin Downie

Introduction

There is a tradition, probably originating in Plato's *Phaedrus*, which depicts the mental state of the creative artist as being akin to that of the madman and the lover.[1] The question raised by this conjunction is whether the creative writer can provide any genuine insights into human behaviour. That is the question I shall try to answer.

In the *Republic* Plato is very clear that creative artists cannot provide any genuine understanding. In Book X of the *Republic* Plato speaks of an 'ancient quarrel' between philosophers (nowadays read 'scientists') and poets and dramatists.[2] The quarrel concerns the qualifications of each to make recommendations on a good or fulfilled or flourishing life. Plato has no doubt that poets and dramatists are trying to do the same kind of thing as the philosophers but believes they are attempting to influence their listeners without having first-hand knowledge and understanding. In fact, he does not think that the poets and dramatists have any proper sort of understanding at all; they are too far removed from the truth. Is Plato correct in thinking that only scientists can provide us with real understanding of human beings, and that creative writers are at best entertainers and at worst downright misleading?

Taking the particular case of our understanding of madness I shall argue that Plato is half right. In many works of creative writing madness is used simply as a literary device, which provides no understanding of the phenomenon but has other literary functions. But he is only half right, because some creative writers have succeeded in providing an understanding of madness which complements that of the scientific psychiatrist. I shall begin by examining some uses of madness as a device, and then move on to my central theme, which is to contrast scientific accounts of madness with those found in some works of literature.

Madness as a literary device

Like other literary devices the use of madness can be successful or unsuccessful in a work, but to the extent that it is just a device it can have the unfortunate side-effect of encouraging stereotypical views of madness. This, of course, supports Plato's thesis that creative writers can be misleading. For example, the case of the first Mrs Rochester in Charlotte Bronte's *Jane Eyre* is one which works successfully in the novel but perpetuates half-truths about madness.[3]

The mad Mrs Rochester is introduced by means of the devices of the Gothic novel. Jane Eyre is taken by Mrs Fairfax up a narrow staircase to the attics, where she hears strange laughter, explained away but not to Jane's satisfaction. Later Jane hears demoniacal laughter. She (daringly) opens the door of her chamber, sees a candle and discovers that Mr Rochester's bedroom has been set on fire. Fear increases when Jane is at her casement looking at the moon and hears a terrible cry. It emerges that Mrs Rochester's brother has been knifed and bitten. Jane is given some information on this but not the whole story. On the eve of her wedding there is another fearful incident. The mad woman enters Jane's bedroom. Her face is described as 'discoloured', 'savage', with rolling red eyes and 'fearful blackened inflation of the lineaments'. This 'Vampyre' takes Jane's wedding veil and 'rent it in two parts, flinging both on the floor...'. The final truth comes out after the wedding is stopped (an incident which has worried brides ever since) and Mr Rochester gives a full account of the matter.

It seems that Mr Rochester was pushed into an ill-considered marriage by his father and elder brother to help the fortunes of the family. The woman in question, Bertha Mason, who, we are told, is a Creole, came of a family in which madness was inherent. But she was also depraved and this seems to have hastened the insanity – 'her excesses had prematurely developed the germs of insanity'. In the end, she is returned to Thornfield Hall and locked up in the attic.

There are several literary ends to which this story of madness is put. First, it gives to the conventional love-story an element of fear. This is skilfully introduced, and is still effective even in our more cynical age. Secondly, it gives the story a dramatic incident, when the wedding is stopped. Again, this is effective because it seems to put paid to Jane's hopes, while not entirely blackening the character of Mr Rochester. Finally, it can be used to bring out the good qualities both in Jane – she tells us (in chapter XXVII) that the unfortunate lady 'cannot help being mad' – and in Mr Rochester. Mr Rochester does not hate Bertha because she is mad – he wouldn't hate Jane if she were mad – but because of her depravities. And in the end he tries to rescue her and the servants when she sets fire to the Hall, and is blinded in the process.

But although the case of Mrs Rochester may be a successful literary device in the novel, in that it makes the plot more exciting and throws into relief various good human qualities, the case perpetuates a number of false beliefs about madness. There is the belief that it is hereditary. This is sometimes but by no means always true. As well, there is the belief that the mad are always violent, whereas only a small proportion of them may be. Finally, there is the belief that madness and moral depravity go together, and although Jane counters this her counter is not so strong as Rochester's assertions. This highly popular novel therefore does not advance our understanding of madness and may indeed reinforce certain misconceptions about it.

Jean Rhys offers a much more subtle account of Mrs Rochester's madness in *Wide Sargasso Sea*.[4] It is more subtle because it places Mrs Rochester in the context of her life-story and historical culture. Charlotte Bronte did not set out to write a novel which would give us any understanding of madness, but Jean Rhys, herself from the West Indies, did set out to redress the balance, to provide an account of Mrs Rochester (Antoinette as she is called in the novel) in the context of life in the West Indies after the emancipation of slaves. The account is convincing because of its complexity and its ambiguity. Jean Rhys shows how a changing cultural context can affect a person's grasp of her identity, and how loss of identity can be a factor in the creation of one kind of madness. I shall later argue that it is a writer's ability to bring out in subtle ways – as in this novel – the layers of meaning in a situation which assists our understanding of a phenomenon such as madness.

William Wordsworth, in his poem *The Idiot Boy*, makes a totally different use of madness.[5] The idiot boy of the poem, Johnny, has some sort of cognitive impairment, and, of course, 'the village idiot' was a common sight in rural England at the time. Johnny is cared for by his mother, Betty Foy, while his father is absent on a woodcutting expedition. Betty encounters what would nowadays be called an 'ethical dilemma'. Her neighbour, Susan Gale, becomes ill and needs immediate attention, and possibly treatment from the local doctor. Betty cannot both go to the assistance of Susan and also fetch the doctor. Her decision is to send Johnny on the back of a very gentle pony for the doctor while she herself goes to nurse Susan. The poem describes the repeated instructions which Johnny is given and the mother's anxiety. While Betty is with Susan she expresses an outward confidence that he will soon return with the doctor, and she devotes all her attention to Susan. But as time passes her anxiety begins to show:

> But yet I guess that now and then
> With Betty all was not so well;
> And to the road she turns her ears,
> And thence full many a sound she hears,
> Which she to Susan will not tell.

Betty would like to go and look for Johnny, but Susan appears to be getting worse. Finally, it is Susan who tells Betty to go and seek Johnny. A long passage brings out the increasing anxieties of Betty as to the fate of Johnny. She reaches the doctor and wakes him. This doctor, I'm afraid, has not attended the ethics classes and does not come out of it very well:

> The Doctor, looking somewhat grim,
> 'What, Woman, should I know of him?'
> And, grumbling, he went back to bed.

Eventually she does see the boy and the pony, ambling along quite unbothered:

> She looks again – her arms are up –
> She screams – she cannot move for joy;
> She darts, as with a torrent's force,
> She almost has o'erturned the Horse,
> And fast she holds her Idiot Boy.

Betty is not at all angry with Johnny but just relieved to have him safe with her again: 'Oh! Johnny, never mind the Doctor;/ You've done your best – and that is all'. Even Susan has recovered from her physical ailment through worrying about the fate of Johnny! Johnny's account of his absence, from eight o'clock in the evening until five in the morning, is just that he has listened to the owls and watched the moon.

What understanding does this poem give us of cognitive impairment? Virtually none! The account of the Idiot Boy is a standard one, of someone not able to concentrate or remember information. So while our feelings for Johnny may be engaged, it cannot really be said that our understanding of mental handicap is advanced. But to see the poem as an attempt to give us some insight into cognitive impairment is to miss the point. The point is not to give us insight into the mental state of Johnny but into the feelings of the mother, and to some extent of her neighbour, Susan.

Wordsworth places the poem along with *Michael* and some others in a group entitled *Poems Founded on the Affections*.[6] And that is the clue to the meaning of the poem. What it does is to give us insight into human feelings, the way in which the overwhelming capacity of the human heart for love can be directed at an impaired human being. We are led to see the glory of human beings as residing not in the triumphs of the intellect but in the overflowing of feeling. This indeed was a common theme in Wordsworth's poetry.

These are just two out of many possible examples of the use of madness as a device in literature. Such uses can be successful as literary devices, but do not advance our understanding of it. It is to the understanding of madness that I shall now turn, beginning with a brief account of what is involved in the scientific understanding of madness. In its brevity, the account will of necessity be crude to the point of parody, but it may serve to make the contrast I hope to bring out.

Scientific understanding and madness

Let us first return to Plato's views on creative writers and the limitations of their attempts to understand the world. Plato's view is that real understanding comes from having insight into the blueprints, the timeless patterns which make things as they are. In our day the task of discovering such patterns has been taken over by the scientists.

We might say that scientists are attempting to trace order, or repeatable patterns, in the apparent randomness of what we observe. These patterns can be anything from the orbits of the planets to the typical development of a tumour. We could put it another way by saying that one way in which the sciences provide understanding is by demonstrating that events, and indeed pieces of organic and non-organic matter, are not endlessly different or individual but can be classified into types. The beginnings of scientific classification can be traced to Aristotle, who distinguished the types into 'genera' and 'species'.[7] For Aristotle, to understand is to be able to classify, to be able to show that there is order in the apparently random; and the better the scientist the more refined the systems of classification. Whereas the terminology has changed a little (say, in botany), Aristotle's approach to the scientific understanding of the world is still accepted, especially in medicine.

The same kind of account can be given of the behavioural sciences. They attempt to provide understanding by tracing patterns in human behaviour. There has been less success here because of the complexity of human behaviour, and the ethical and practical problems which arise through any attempt to experiment on human behaviour. Nevertheless, the principle is the same: the behavioural sciences, like the natural sciences, attempt to provide understanding through tracing repeatable patterns, the types of behaviour shown by the manic-depressive or indeed by a normal person who is dying. In a longer account of patterns something would need to be said about the related idea of the repeatable elements in nature and their connection with generalisations or laws, and predictability. But these would be developments rather than additions to the basic point.

There is a second, although connected, way in which the sciences try to give us understanding of the world, and that is through discovering the underlying causality of the patterns. For example, an early botanist might have observed that insectivorous plants, such as butterwort, typically grow in boggy terrains. The more modern biochemically-minded botanist could explain the pattern by establishing that a boggy terrain is deficient in nitrogen and that the plant obtains nitrogen by ingesting insects. Thus the pattern is explained in terms of an underlying causality. Once again the same is true of behaviour patterns. An early scientist such as Hippocrates noted the behaviour patterns which are typical of epilepsy, say, while a modern scientist would try to explain such patterns in terms of the underlying causality of the brain.

These two characteristics of scientific explanation are to be found also in scientific accounts of madness. For example, a psychiatrist will record the behaviour patterns which are typical of certain sorts of neurosis or psychosis. Perhaps more accurately he will note certain abnormal behaviour patterns and name these in terms of the classificatory language of psychiatry. Thus, the manic-depressive or the schizophrenic will typically exhibit certain behaviour patterns, and a patient displaying some or all of these will be appropriately classified. Some scientific understanding of madness, then, is created when the psychiatrist can identify and label the behaviour pattern which the patient is exhibiting. The psychiatrist in research mode, however, will not be content with classification, but will seek the underlying causality of such patterns. Is there a biochemical imbalance? Is there some decay of brain cells? Have there been disturbing events in childhood?

It is worth noting that, although the modern psychiatrist is much more sophisticated than Plato in his explanations of madness, the type of understanding he attempts to provide is no different in principle from that which Plato attempts to provide. Plato sees the behaviour of a person who possesses mental health as balanced. The different elements of the mind – desires, emotions and reason – are in harmony, and this harmony stems from an underlying harmony in the elements of the body. Madness, for Plato, occurs when the normal equilibrium is disturbed, and in particular when reason is no longer in charge. He is a little afraid that this is what happens not only to the straightforwardly mad but also to poets and lovers. Perhaps he is right.

A rather similar account of mental health and mental illness is given by Freud:

> The mental apparatus is composed of an 'id' which is the repository of the instinctual elements, of an 'ego' which is the most superficial portion of the id and one which has been modified by the influences of the external world, and of a 'superego' which develops out of the ego, and represents the inhibitions of instinct which are characteristic of man.[8]

Freud is here offering a tri-partite view of the psyche rather similar to that of Plato. Moreover, he goes on, again in a manner similar to Plato, to regard mental health as harmony between the parts of the soul, and mental illness as unresolved conflict between them.

There are many similar contemporary accounts of mental health and mental illness, sometimes using a word like 'equilibrium' as a scientific-sounding equivalent of Plato's 'harmony'. The different types of disequilibrium can be classified as the different types of mental illness. What all these accounts have in common is an attempt to generalise, to say something which is true of all species of mental illness. This kind of project is characteristic of both the scientist and the philosopher. It is the attempt to find a pattern, or a blueprint, of mental illness or of madness, and then to find the causal structure underlying that pattern.

There is a third feature of the scientific approach which we might term 'reductivism'. The term is used in a variety of ways, but what I have in mind here is the tendency to treat the phenomenon to be explained in isolation from its total context. The origins of this tendency can be seen in early modern physics where the laws of moving bodies, for example, are investigated and established in isolation from other factors such as air resistance. To the extent that the behavioural sciences modelled themselves on the natural sciences this tendency is also found in them. This reductivist tendency is encouraged because reductivism makes it easier to assign numbers to the phenomena being explained, and numbers give the appearance (often deceptive) of objectivity and rigour.

A fourth characteristic of scientific understanding concerns the scientific attitude. This characteristic can best be identified if we take an example. Suppose a psychiatrist is interviewing a patient and the patient becomes angry and abusive. The response of the psychiatrist will be detached in the sense that she will not take personally anything said, but rather will interpret the anger as the result of causal forces the patient cannot control; the anger will be seen as a symptom. Suppose now that the same psychiatrist later in the day encounters anger from the Chief Executive of the hospital trust. Let us say that she has parked her car in the Chief Executive's space. In this case she will respond differently, perhaps with indignation, 'There was no other space and I was called in urgently to see a case', or perhaps with embarrassment, 'I'm sorry, I just didn't notice that it was exclusively your space'. But however the psychiatrist responds, the general nature of the response will be essentially different from that which she offers to the patient. Some philosophers have contrasted the 'objective' attitude, when we respond to deeds and words as to the effects of causes, with the 'reactive' attitude, when we assume that deeds and words have a human meaning and are to be taken at their face value as parts of ordinary human interaction.[9] We might say that the distinction is between the scientifically or technically or professionally detached, where the interest terminates in the phenomenon in question, and the humane, where there is a deeper resonance involving human feelings.

Well-known lines in Wordsworth's poem *Peter Bell* illustrate the point here:

> A primrose by a river's brim
> A yellow primrose was to him
> It was nothing more.[10]

Or more tellingly in the parody:

> A primrose by a river's brim
> Dicotyledon was to him,
> It was nothing more.

A fifth feature of the scientific approach to understanding, like the fourth, characterises the professional scientific attitude; it concerns the absence of any value judgements which the psychiatrist might make on the patient. The psychiatrist is concerned only with the fact that the behaviour pattern or the thoughts and words of the patient are either socially damaging or may lead to self-destruction. The thoughts, words, or deeds of the patient are abnormal in the sense that they deviate from what is the social norm of the society at the time, or they prevent the patient from doing what he/she might want to do, or what a 'normal' person of that society might want to do. This fifth aspect of the scientific approach to understanding we might think of as the 'non-judgemental' approach and it means something like 'neutral with respect to values'.

So far I have suggested that the scientific understanding of madness has five (perhaps overlapping) characteristics: it requires the discovery of patterns, underlying causality, and it is reductivist; and it requires professional detachment and value neutrality. If that were the only mode of understanding then we would need to agree with Plato that the arts cannot give us real understanding of madness, or indeed of anything else. For literary writing lacks the five features I have identified. But I shall try to show that there are other modes of understanding which a creative writer can offer, and that these are relevant to the understanding of madness.

Literary understanding and madness

How can we understand something if not by discovering the kind of pattern into which it fits? One possible way is in terms of a type of formation other than a pattern – namely, a sequence. Patterns are a-temporal and, as it were, they structure space. An example is the double-helix which is the pattern of the DNA molecule. But events and human actions follow each other in time. This gives us a sequence, and a sequence structures time. This suggests another type of understanding: we can be shown how a person's action might fit in to the unique sequence which is their life. For example, we might ask why Mr A, who lives next door and is known to dislike gardening, has spent all weekend working in his garden, and we might come to understand when we are told that he is putting his house on the market and thinks it will sell better with a tidy garden. The first point here is that we can now see the action in the sequence of events and actions which constitute Mr A's life. Secondly, there are explicit and implicit references to individual and social purposes and values such as selling houses and keeping gardens tidy. These are familiar to us and for that reason relating Mr A's actions to them helps our understanding. Thirdly, because such purposes and values are ones which those who are in a certain social context can share, and with which they can have a sympathetic identification, understanding is deepened. Fourthly, the story of Mr A implies a variety of standpoints. There are hints of curious neighbours, perhaps disapproving of the untidy garden, of speculation about Mr A's motivation and so on. Our understanding involves a complex mixture of individual purposes, social norms, and contrasted viewpoints. In a word, it is holistic.

The points are better illustrated by stories on a grander scale, such as those offered by a biographer or a historian or a novelist. The kind of understanding created by such literary works has become fashionable at the moment in medical circles and more widely. It is sometimes called 'narrative' understanding because it is the sort of understanding which we can obtain from a story. Perhaps in reaction to the current emphasis on 'evidence-based medicine' there has been a new awareness that patients' stories about themselves, their anecdotes, can be relevant to their diagnosis and treatment.[11] Indeed, it can be maintained that it is in terms of our stories about ourselves, and also our emotions and future projects, that our very identity as persons consists. The identity of a person, it might be argued, is more like that of a drama than like that of a material object. To maintain this is really to maintain two points: that we have a serial identity and that we have an individual identity. Just as the play *Hamlet* has a serial identity through time, and a different one from *Macbeth*, so we all have our own unique identities unfolding through time. As we have already seen, Jean Rhys treats the way an increasing confusion about her cultural and individual identity caused the first Mrs Rochester to decline into madness.

This account suggests that we have identified an important kind of understanding which cannot be provided by the sciences but can be provided by the arts. Moreover, understanding can be assisted if our emotions are engaged and we can identify with someone's situation: we are enabled to appreciate their values, and how these values might derive from or contrast with those prevailing in their culture. To develop these abstract points I shall now take some examples of the ways in which great writers have used this method of giving us understanding of a particular sort of madness.

The first example is that of Septimus Warren Smith in Virginia Woolf's novel *Mrs Dalloway*.[12] Septimus is introduced to us in the middle of other events. Mrs Dalloway has been buying sweet peas in Bond Street for her party when a large car with blinds on the windows draws in to the pavement. Passers-by stop and speculate about the important passengers in the car. In the middle of this inconsequential scene Septimus Warren Smith is introduced: he too is unable to pass because everything and everybody has stopped. We are given a description of Septimus:

> ...aged about thirty, pale-faced, beak-nosed, wearing brown shoes, and a shabby overcoat, with hazel eyes which had that look of apprehension in them which makes complete strangers apprehensive too.[13]

The description is significant but is tucked in amidst a scene resembling an Impressionist painting: old ladies on tops of buses with black, red and green parasols against the heat, Mrs Dalloway with her arms full of sweet peas. This charming description is disturbed again when the theme of the apprehension in Septimus's eyes is developed and he is depicted as seeing the bright colours becoming flames and as feeling responsible for blocking the way. He feels rooted to the pavement and everyone is looking at him. We feel something is badly wrong here, and sympathise with his Italian wife, Lucrezia, when she moves him on. With a nice touch we see the complexity of her feelings: she is worried and embarrassed by his behaviour, but cannot help looking at the car too and speculating about its occupants. Ordinary human reactions can be present in the middle of worrying events. The scene introducing Septimus and his problems, then merges with the bustling activity of Bond Street, further speculation about the occupant of the car, perhaps the Queen, and an aeroplane overhead trailing a smoke advertisement for toffee. The first step in assisting us in our understanding of Septimus has been taken, in that our interest and our sympathies have been engaged, and the problems of Septimus have been placed in the value-framework of a total social context.

Septimus appears again a little later when he and Lucrezia have reached Regent's Park, and she draws his attention to the aeroplane. This gives the author a context for telling us that Septimus has already been attending a doctor, for Dr Holmes has recommended to Lucrezia that Septimus be encouraged to take an interest in things outside himself. But he stares fixedly at the smoke trail and is not diverted by it. Lucrezia is embarrassed and walks off a little by herself, and via her thoughts we learn that Septimus has threatened to kill himself. But despite the views of Dr Holmes he is not a coward, for he fought bravely in the war.

In this passage we are told a bit more of the story of Septimus, but also we feel the isolation of Lucrezia. She cannot understand his behaviour, and she can tell no one about her worries. Her isolation is made worse because she is in an alien country. In a subsequent episode we learn of the young Septimus in love with Miss Isabella Pole who lectured on Shakespeare, and of his boss who approved of his work in the auctioneer's but wanted to make a man of him. Septimus volunteered, and with understated bitterness Virginia Woolf tells us that in the trenches in France manliness developed. Septimus was promoted and became very friendly with his officer, Evans. Then we learn that Evans was killed, and that Septimus felt very little about it at the time. But he began to have moments of fear, and found a refuge in the company of the daughters of the innkeeper in Milan where he was billetted. After the war he is welcomed back to his firm as a hero. Then in assorted contexts we are led to see the seriousness of his problems: sexual problems, loathing of other human beings, and self-loathing. Finally, he is persuaded to see Dr Holmes, who is described in a very unattractive manner, perhaps reflecting Virginia Woolf's own experiences of doctors. The scene ends in a very worrying way because Septimus is now hearing Evans speaking, and Dr Holmes recommends a Harley Street specialist, Sir William Bradshaw. Our understanding has deepened because we have learned more of the biography of Septimus and the history of the time. It is also worth noting that this kind of understanding can proceed in tandem with scientific explanation, for there are at least hints of the classification and causality of this type of madness.

Sir William Bradshaw prescribes that Septimus should be taken to a home. Interestingly enough, Sir William's view of mental health and illness is precisely the one we have seen in Plato – harmony or equilibrium, which he calls 'proportion':

> Worshipping proportion, Sir William not only prospered himself but made England prosper, secluded her lunatics, forbade childbirth, penalised despair, made it impossible for the unfit to propagate their views until they, too, shared his sense of proportion – his, if they were men, Lady Bradshaw's if they were women.[14]

In the long final scene there is a faint ray of light in the gathering darkness. Septimus briefly seems more like himself, and jokes and helps design a hat for Lucrezia. She is on his side. But then she tells him he must go to Bradshaw's home, 'must' because he threatened to kill himself. When Holmes finally arrives to take him away Lucrezia tries to block Holmes' approach but he forces himself in. Septimus is poised on the window sill and throws himself on to the railings.

Now of course I have been obliged to omit many of the details of this account of developing madness, but perhaps I have provided enough to enable me to make some general comments. First, by means of a story which gradually unfolds, we come to understand something of the condition which Septimus has got into. That story is part of a complex tapestry of events in the novel. Moreover, we can see the problem from several points of view. From that of Septimus we understand how he has come to feel a hatred for human beings because of the events he was part of in the war, and we see that he has developed a hatred of himself because he feels responsible for the events and especially for the death of his friend Evans. This story is set against other trivial incidents in London which have the effect of sharpening the poignancy of the unfolding story. But we also see the case from the points of view of others and especially from that of Lucrezia, who fills in details of the story of Septimus and provides a set of reactions. The case of Septimus then is a good account of the sequential understanding which we can acquire from a quasi-biography with its assorted value standpoints and social context. There is no attempt to generalise, or to fit the case of Septimus into that of other shell-shock cases. It may be a typical case, but our understanding is of the specific case of Septimus because it is with that case that we identify.

We should note too that the author does not ignore hints about the causality of the madness. Obviously the events of the war are shown to be the major factors, but also we learn that Septimus has a sensitive nature, that he feels guilty about Evans, and that he feels guilty about marrying Lucrezia, whom he did not love. Nothing much is made of these causal factors because the stress is on a different kind of understanding via the total narrative.

Turning now to the attitude we are encouraged to adopt to Septimus and the events in his life, we find that instead of the attitude of scientific detachment other aids to understanding are used. We the readers are not detached from the story of Septimus but enter into his situation. We are made to feel his horror of the shells and the death of his friend; we can share his loathing of the human race; like him we can fear and detest Holmes and Bradshaw. But we are also brought to share the feelings and the point of view of Lucrezia. In a word, we are involved in the unfolding story.

Value judgements also are everywhere implicit in the story, and they assist our understanding of the growing madness. But the value judgements are complex. The war, the main causal factor in the madness, is certainly deplored – 'school boys with gunpowder'.[15] It should be noted that the condemnation of the war in that bitter phrase brings out a huge amount about the English society which created that war – the misplaced (public) school boy attitudes, the patriotism, the lack of grasp about what would be involved, and so on. The upper class social attitudes of the time are also deplored when they masquerade as medical knowledge – outside interests, cricket, not too much Shakespeare, a sense of proportion and so on. The value judgements are always subtle and subtly expressed. From one point of view Clarissa Dalloway is a silly rich woman, but yet we can understand the values of her life, and we note that she comes to condemn Sir William

Bradshaw. The attitude that we are encouraged to adopt towards Sir William Bradshaw can be detected in other novels of madness. For example, in Wilkie Collins' novel *The Woman in White* we are shown the powerlessness of the individual against 'expert' medical opinion.[16] The tensions produced by this tapestry of varied values are an aid to our understanding of the specific case of Septimus.

But our understanding does not terminate with the case of Septimus. By means of that story of developing madness we come to understand a total social context. It points beyond itself and becomes a symbol of something much deeper. It enriches our human perceptions of ourselves and of a historical period. Even more than that, it reaches what is universal in the human condition through the exploration of the particular case. To stress this kind of understanding is not at all to denigrate the attempts of psychiatrists and others to understand the phenomena of madness and shellshock in particular; no doubt numerical generalisations of types of case have their important place. But I wish to make a plea for the kind of understanding which comes from literature, an understanding in which the reader can move from a total involvement with an individual case in its full context to something universal.

Shakespeare is another writer who gives us insight into different types of madness, interestingly before scientific accounts existed. Moreover, he distinguishes madness of different kinds brought on by a variety of circumstances in *Macbeth, Hamlet* and *King Lear*. I shall take just one example.

In *King Lear* we find a very complex study of madness, involving Lear himself, the simulated madness of Edgar, and the commentary of the Fool.[17] The different sorts of madness are judged against a running discussion of what it is 'natural' to do, and what it is reasonable to do. We are warned that the seeds of madness have always been there in Lear. Regan reminds Goneril: "Tis the infirmity of his age: yet he hath ever but slenderly known himself' (Act I, scene I, lines 292–93). The events of the play exacerbate this condition. At the start we have a display of embarrassing senility – behaviour which, while it is not mad, is certainly perceived as contrary to natural reason and sentiment. Lear is depicted as having a traditional hierarchical outlook of which his behaviour represents the pathology. Goneril and Regan, on the other hand, come from another way of looking at what is reasonable; for them the reasonable is the pursuit of rational self-interest and the only sentiment they recognise as having a claim is the satisfaction of the desires of the self. The tragedy of the play is the collision of these two ways of looking at the world, and Lear's madness is the outcome of that collision. He cannot understand how what he considers to be the natural sentiments of love for a parent and deference to authority can be so ignored by his own daughters. But with his madness comes insight. He sees the harsher side of the world order he represents and, spurred on by the Fool, he comes to see his own failings, and those of all of us.

It is interesting that Virginia Woolf suffered from recurring bouts of mental illness, and finally took her own life. Plato argues that the suspected madness of artists (and lovers) disqualifies them from making claims to real understanding of human beings. But he may be wrong here, for it is plausible that in the case of Virginia Woolf (and she is just one of many possible examples from the arts) it is the mental ill-health which is the source of the insight. More generally, it is true that to achieve a sympathetic insight into another person's life and problems it is necessary to be a certain sort of person. Literature (and other arts) can be of assistance in that kind of personal development. Medical educationists take note!

Some critics may object that a sympathetic biographical understanding, as opposed to scientific understanding, has the huge disadvantage that it cannot give rise to treatment. But this is not wholly true. Patients may have stories about themselves and their lives, but people are not fixed by their stories. It is possible to persuade someone to see their life in a different way, to stress the more positive side to it. We do this with our friends, and it is possible also in clinical practice. There can be talking cures as well as drug cures.

Finally, it should be noted that the two sorts of understanding I have outlined are compatible. We can understand another person in more than one way.

Conclusion

In this somewhat breathless survey of the many ways in which madness has been used in literature I have tried to show that it can be both a literary device and also a means of providing understanding and insights into madness which are complementary to scientific accounts. I have of course said nothing about other ways in which madness appears in literature. For example, I have said nothing about a familiar literary figure, 'the mad scientist', or about madness in novels or other works which campaign for a change in the law or a more tolerant attitude. My central themes have been that, as a device, the use of madness can be more or less successful in a plot, and it can also serve to symbolise extreme aspects of human nature, or more crudely to trigger emotions such as fear. But creative writing can also provide a kind of understanding of or a new perspective on madness which can stand beside that of the psychiatrist.

Notes

1 Plato, 'Phaedrus', *The Collected Dialogues of Plato*, ed. Edith Hamilton and Huntington Cairns (New York, 1963), pp. 475–525.
2 Plato, 'The Republic', *Dialogues of Plato*, Book X, 607b, p. 832.
3 Charlotte Brontë, *Jane Eyre*, ed. Michael Mason (Harmondsworth, 1996).
4 Jean Rhys, *Wide Sargasso Sea* (Harmondsworth, 1968).

5 William Wordsworth, 'The Idiot Boy', *Poetical Works*, ed. Ernest de Selincourt (Oxford, 1981), pp. 100–104.

6 Wordsworth, 'Poems Founded on the Affections', *Poetical Works*, pp. 100–121.

7 Aristotle, 'Metaphysics', *The Basic Works of Aristotle*, ed. Richard McKeon (New York, 1941), 1037–1039, pp. 802–806.

8 Sigmund Freud, *The Standard Edition of the Complete Psychological Works of Sigmund Freud*, ed. James Strachey (London, 1953–74), vol. 20, p. 201.

9 John Macmurray, *Persons in Relation*, vol 2 of *The Form of the Personal* (London, 1961), pp. 28–31; Peter Strawson, 'Freedom and Resentment', *Freedom and Resentment and Other Essays* (London, 1974), pp. 1–26.

10 Wordsworth, 'Peter Bell', *Poetical Works*, pp. 188–198.

11 R. S. Downie and Jane Macnaughton, *Clinical Judgement: Evidence in Practice* (Oxford, 2000), pp. 51–60.

12 Virginia Woolf, *Mrs Dalloway* (London, 1982).

13 Woolf, *Mrs Dalloway*, p. 14.

14 Woolf, *Mrs Dalloway*, p. 15.

15 Woolf, *Mrs Dalloway*, p. 86.

16 Wilkie Collins, *The Woman in White*, ed. Matthew Sweet (Harmondsworth, 1999), p. 434.

17 William Shakespeare, *King Lear*, ed. G. K. Hunter (Harmondsworth, 1972).

Part II

Madness in Literature:
Medieval to Modern

4
'The thoghtful maladie': Madness and Vision in Medieval Writing

Corinne Saunders

Shoshana Felman has written, 'To speak about madness is to speak about the difference between languages: to import into one language the strangeness of another; to unsettle the decisions language has prescribed to us so that, somewhere between languages, will emerge the freedom to speak'.[1] Speaking 'about madness' need not exclusively mean as a psychiatrist, a literary critic or a historian of ideas. Those who have experienced some form of what they or their contemporaries term madness or mental illness are often impelled – or inspired – perhaps as part of the process to recovery, to speak of it, to import into everyday language that strangeness. A key question is whether madness should be seen as providing a subject about which to write, or instead as in some way inspiring artistic creativity. This essay will argue that both perspectives are valid: the 'freedom to speak' that Felman describes may be the result both of the desire to speak *about* and to speak *from* that otherness of madness. This is exemplified with special clarity in the writing of the Middle Ages, a period of acute awareness of madness as not only threatening and absolute in its otherness but also as a state of potential grace.

The link between madness and creativity is as old as western literature. For the Greeks, poetry was a healing art: the Greek god Apollo was the patron both of poetry and medicine. Poetry was seen as possessing the power to heal, not only its audience, but the poet himself. Pindar, in the *Pythian Odes*, writes:

> He is the god who sends
> mortal men and women
> relief from grievous disease, Apollo,
> who has given us the lyre,
> who brings the Muse
> to whom he chooses, filling the heart
> with peace and harmony'.[2]

Aristotle's theory of *katharsis* works similarly. The poet occupied a special status: paradoxically, his healing inspiration was viewed as something closely associated with possession or madness, for it opened onto the realms of the divine and irrational. In Plato's *Ion*, Socrates persuades the rhapsode that his poetry is the result not of reason and learning, but of divine inspiration or madness:

> For the authors of those great poems which we admire, do not attain to excellence through the rules of any art, but they utter their beautiful melodies of verse in a state of inspiration, and, as it were, possessed by a spirit not their own. Thus the composers of lyrical poetry create those admired songs of theirs in a state of divine insanity....
>
> ...
>
> For a Poet is indeed a thing ethereally light, winged, and sacred, nor can he compose anything worth calling poetry until he becomes inspired, and, as it were, mad, or whilst any reason remains in him.[3]

In the *Phaedrus*, Plato identifies 'the third type of possession and madness' as 'possession by the Muses', making a similar point, 'if a man comes to the door of poetry untouched by the madness of the Muses, believing that technique alone will make him a good poet, he and his sane compositions never reach perfection, but are utterly eclipsed by the performances of the inspired madman'.[4] In the same way, Plato tells us in the *Timaeus*, 'inspired and true prophecy' can only occur 'when the power of our understanding is inhibited by sleep, or we are in an abnormal condition owing to disease or divine inspiration': it is associated with the 'irrational part' of the soul situated in the liver.[5] In Plato's *Republic* the poet is forbidden in the ideal city, for he 'destroys the reasonable part' of the soul; 'he is a maker of images which are very far removed from the truth'.[6] Poetry is seen as a divine frenzy, and while this may be an extreme view, western thought and literature through the Middle Ages and beyond very much retain the idea of madness (and to some extent illness more generally) as a heightened state that opens the way for the creative act, a state of intensity in which the sufferer is taken out of himself, paradoxically to come to a new state of self-realisation or understanding of the world around him. Michel Foucault memorably captures such a state in speaking of 'the lyric glow of illness'.[7]

Foucault identifies the eighteenth century as the great period of change in attitudes to madness, the period of the asylum, when the mad are shut away from the world. While, as Roy Porter has noted, the notion of an absolute shift in ideas from one period to another can be dangerously monolithic, it is reasonable to characterise the Middle Ages as distinct from later periods, in that madness was of necessity more a part of the everyday world.[8] There were almost no hospitals where the mentally ill could be treated, so that these people were part of the community, cared for by family or servants; the likelihood of any cure was small.[9] Madness was viewed as an aspect of God's providential patterning of the universe, mysteriously sent to light on particular individuals, perhaps as a test or a punishment, and sometimes as mysteriously, miraculously, removed. In the Middle Ages any connection made between madness and creativity is shaped by a strong sense of the divine will underlying the experience of madness. Crucial too is the identification of passion with the realms of the irrational. Thus there was admiration as well as condemnation for some kinds of 'madness', and the line between madness and religious vision was blurred.

What did 'madness' mean in medieval England? It has sometimes been assumed that madness was exclusively equated with demonic possession, and that all those manifesting signs of mental illness were regarded as witches, likely to be put to death; in fact, the witch trials occurred later, in the early modern period.[10] The possibility of demonic possession was taken seriously by medieval writers, and from the Bible onwards there existed numerous accounts of demonic possession. In Gregory the Great's *Dialogues*, written in the sixth century and translated into English by King Alfred's bishop Wærferth, we find the memorable story of a nun who carelessly bit into a lettuce without crossing herself first and was immediately possessed, 'þa wearð heo sona fram deofle ʒeʒripen & niðer on þa eorðan ʒefeoll & wæs swiþe ʒeswenced' ('Then immediately she was gripped by the devil, and fell down onto the ground and was very greatly tormented'). The devil, when challenged by the holy abbot, complains, '"hwæt dyde ic hire? hwæt dyde ic hire? ic me sæt on anum leahtrice, þa com heo & bat me"' ('"what did I do to her? what did I do to her? I was sitting on a lettuce, when she came and bit me."').[11] The story is comic, but captures the sense of the devil as always lurking nearby, ready to invade the human body. Other narratives of possession described not only what were evidently cases of epilepsy, but also instances of 'psychiatric syndrome[s] of possession', of individuals apparently taken over by 'an alien personality', speaking in different voices or manifesting changes in thought and behaviour. Robert Louis Stevenson's *The Strange Case of Dr Jekyll and Mr Hyde* (1886) provides the most celebrated literary example, but by no means the first.[12] Some of the cases recorded may have been cases of schizophrenia, multiple personality disorder, or Tourette's syndrome, where the sufferer may compulsively manifest tics or speak obscenities. The inexplicability and strangeness of such conditions intersected with a readiness to believe in the possibility of demonic possession, whether as a result of innate human weakness, as punishment for sin, as a form of testing, or as an element of the devil's great plan to cause the downfall of mankind. If, as philosophers such as Aquinas argued, the devil could possess the bodies of sleeping women to beget changeling children, he could also invade the human body in other ways; the New Testament provided ample exemplification of demonic possession.

It is striking, however, that while theological works are likely to include numerous accounts of demonic possession, medical treatises focus on physiological explanations for madness.

Possession was, however, by no means seen as the only cause of madness. Medical thought in this period was shaped by the theory of the four bodily humours, developed by Hippocrates and Galen, and influential up to the nineteenth century. The four humours, each associated with a bodily fluid, reflected the division of nature into four elements: the exact makeup of the humours created an individual's temperament and complexion.[13] Ideally, this comprised a balance of humours; imbalance created illness. This theory meant that the modern distinction between physical and mental illness did not exist (though it is interesting that recent medical thought has come to emphasise anew the mind-body continuum): in the Middle Ages, all illnesses were viewed as physiological, rooted in some imbalance of the humours. Since humours were seen as shaping individual temperaments, it seemed unsurprising that their disorder was seen as potentially affecting the mind as well as the body.

Some effort was made in medieval medicine to go beyond these broad ideas, and thus different types of mental illness were associated with different parts of the brain. Four main mental disorders were distinguished: melancholy, mania, phrenitis and epilepsy.[14] Most important was melancholy (caused by an excess of black bile), which probably included the diseases now classified as depression, schizophrenia and paranoia, and which was often seen as the origin of other mental disorders. Melancholy was characterised by fear or suspicion, and by sadness of an enduring nature, sometimes by sleeplessness or hallucinations, or by atypical social behaviour, whether withdrawal from society or fear of being alone. By the later Middle Ages, melancholy was seen as 'a disorder affecting the cogitative or reasoning power in the central ventricle'.[15] For the modern reader, Hamlet has become the archetypal sufferer of melancholy, and Shakespeare exploits the blurred line between the melancholy humour and madness. By contrast mania, the result of an excess of yellow bile, affected the imagination in the front cerebral ventricle. It was, of course, not always easy to distinguish between diseases of reason and imagination, and in fact melancholy and mania were often simply treated as 'madness'. That the terms were familiar ones, however, is shown in Chaucer's *Knight's Tale*, in which he speaks of mania as stemming from melancholy and attacking the imagination, 'manye / Engendred of humour malencolik / Biforen, in his celle fantastik'.[16] Some writers also distinguished lethargy as a separate disorder that impaired the memory, situated in the rear ventricle. The third main type of madness was 'phrenitis' (a term from which the modern word 'frenzy' derives), a temporary 'disorder characterised by mental derangement and fever'. This kind of violent delirium, believed to be caused by yellow bile on the brain, was perhaps symptomatic of the diseases of meningitis or typhoid fever, rather than mental illness. Epilepsy was also assumed to be a mental illness, and the disorder most likely to be viewed as demonic possession, although medical theory from Hippocrates onwards attributed epilepsy either to phlegm or bile moving to the brain, or to a blockage of the ventricles by these fluids. It seems probable that academic theories of mental disease were held alongside folk beliefs in 'lunacy', the effect of the phases of the moon on the mind, and a popular acceptance of the possibility of demonic possession.

Treatments of mental illness, like the theories of their causes, were not clear cut and were limited, but they did exist: most drastic were the treatments of phlebotomy and bloodletting, performed in order to let the surfeit humours escape.[17] Physicians also prescribed diet, exercise and alterations to surroundings or air, music, art and reading, and, most of all, herbal remedies, not so different, perhaps, from the prescription of St John's Wort now. Patients could be restrained, and occasionally other operations on the skull were performed. There also existed a wide range of magical and folk cures: charms, spells, potions. The mysterious nature of mental illness and the difficulty of treatment meant that 'academic' treatments often overlapped with those rooted in superstition and folk belief. Unsurprisingly, much refuge was sought in religious observances: the Lord might as easily alleviate illness as he sent it, and as mysteriously. Some shrines came to be specially associated with the mentally ill, who might make or be remembered in pilgrimages to them: most famous was the Belgian shrine of Saint Dymphna, patron saint of the insane, who had been killed by her father when she refused to marry him.[18] As well, sufferers and their families or friends might have recourse to holy relics, prayer, and sometimes exorcism.

It is clear that there were academic, medical, theological and popular strands of the medieval dialogue surrounding 'madness' in its various forms. The law too had its own discourse on madness.[19] Madness was legally recognised, and the mentally ill were legally absolved from some responsibility, for they were seen as having lost the power to control the mind. The thirteenth-century legal treatise attributed to Bracton puts this case forcefully, though other medieval legal theorists were less sympathetic:

> But what shall we say of a madman bereft of reason? And of the deranged, the delirious and the mentally retarded? ... *Quare* whether such a one commits a felony *de se* [if he commits suicide]. It is submitted that he does not, nor do such persons forfeit their inheritance or their chattels, since they are without sense and reason and can no more commit ... a felony than a brute animal'.[20]

There is some evidence that crimes committed by the deranged were punished by imprisonment rather than death.[21] By the thirteenth century, the care of the estates of those mentally ill from birth, referred to as 'idiots' or 'natural fools', was given to the king; those who became 'lunatics' (their mental incapacity probably ascertained through simple tests of numbers or memory) were put in the care of private guardians.[22] Institutionalisation was not usually an option: on the Continent, the mentally ill were housed in only a few hospitals, such as the Hotel Dieu in Paris; the first dedicated mental hospital was built in Valencia in 1409. In late fourteenth-century England, the hospital of St Mary of Bethlem ('Bedlam') had space for just 6 patients, providing chains and manacles for them.[23]

While different discourses brought different emphases to the consideration of madness, they share, as Simon Kemp has pointed out, a common definition of madness as 'the inability of the mind, the rational soul, to control behaviour'; there was therefore a strong sense in the Middle Ages of madness as illness, whether caused by physiological imbalance or demonic influence, or both.[24] In madness, man returned to the state of a wild beast, subject to his passions. In the medieval imagination, this was indeed always a danger, for the order of the human psyche was understood to be frail. It was a theological commonplace that before the Fall, man had been governed absolutely by the will: sexual instincts, it was argued, had existed, but only as occasioned by the will, in order to conceive children; the will controlled both the emotions and the mind, including the faculties of imagination and reason. The result of the Fall, when man had succumbed to irrational desire, was concupiscence, the disorder of these faculties. Penelope Doob notes that Hildegarde of Bingen also argued that the Fall 'led to the creation of the melancholy humour, that chief fount of madness and disease'.[25] Fallen man was seen as the site of conflicting emotions, instincts, reason and desires, and the will as perpetually struggling to control these and direct them towards good. The disorder of sexual desire reflected a more general disorder. In this fallen state, it was always possible that the individual should lose control of the will, sometimes altogether, succumbing to madness. Individuals might experience short periods of madness, in which they became the victims of their 'ungoverned passion'; such madness 'might increase to the point of becoming an incurable disease of the soul'.[26]

In medieval writing, madness is frequently portrayed as the result of extreme sinfulness. This is exemplified in John Gower's *Confessio Amantis*, a treatise on the seven deadly sins in relation to love, which collects together a vast number of classical and Biblical stories. The loss of reason again and again characterises those who succumb to sin. Thus in his consideration of the sin of theft or robbery, Gower narrates the story of the rape of Philomela by Tereus, who comes to seem a wild beast, a 'tyrant raviner' without 'Reason – the faculty [that] ... separated man from brute beasts'.[27] The most celebrated medieval example of madness in which man reverts to bestiality is that of Nebuchadnezzar, punished for his sin of pride by his transformation to a bestial state in the wilderness, the landscape viewed in this period as the appropriate domain of the wild or mad man or woman.[28] Gower plays on this association in describing Nebuchadnezzar's fall:

> And thus was he from his kingdom
> Into the wilde Forest drawe
> Wher that the myhti goddes lawe
> Thurgh his pouer dede him transforme
> From man into a bestes forme;
> And lich an Oxe under the fot
> He graseth, as he nedes mot
> To geten him his lives fode. (I, 2968–75)

Gower also elaborates Nebuchadnezzar's gradual return to grace, and recognition of the sinfulness for which he has been punished, describing his growing self-awareness, the distinguishing characteristic of man: 'Upon himself tho gan he loke'; he sees 'In stede of man a bestes lyke (likeness)', and he weeps, praying to heaven 'in his bestly stevene (voice)' (I, 2992, 2995, 3025). The narrative offers a literal exemplification of the association between madness and the bestial state: Nebuchadnezzar actually becomes a beast, transformed back into man's form when he repents and prays.

This association between madness, sinfulness and the bestial recurs on more or less symbolic levels across medieval literature. Even in the seventeenth century, Robert Burton in the *Anatomy of Melancholy* would be definite about this connection:

> ... that which crucifies us most, is our own folly, madness (Whom Jupiter would destroy, he first drives mad; by subtraction of his assisting grace God permits it), weakness, want of government, our facility and proneness in yielding to several lusts, in giving way to every passion and perturbation of the mind: by which means we metamorphose ourselves and degenerate into beasts....

> ... we, as long as we are ruled by reason, correct our inordinate appetites, and conform ourselves to God's word, are as so many living saints: but if we give reins to lust, anger, ambition, pride, and follow our own ways, we degenerate into beasts, transform ourselves, overthrow our constitutions, provoke God to anger, and heap upon us this [affliction] of Melancholy, and all kinds of incurable diseases, as a just and deserved punishment of our sins'.[29]

In a world where illness seemed so inexplicable but so obviously god-sent, perhaps as punishment, and where loss of reason seemed to reflect the passional disorder of the Fall and thus to be linked to a state of sin, a moral view of madness was almost inevitable.

And yet, strikingly, the identification of madness with sin was by no means the only way of understanding mental illness in this period. In the instance of Tereus, evil does indeed manifest itself in madness, and his descent into savage bestiality is in no way creative: rather, it presents a stark moral lesson and warning to the audience. But even the related example of Nebuchadnezzar is more complex in that madness here is also associated with redemption. Nebuchadnezzar's descent into savagery leads to prayer and penance, to the voicing of his sinful human state and self-realisation. This notion of madness as a process of penance or suffering that in some way brings enlightenment can also take other forms: it may not occur as a punishment for an extreme state of sin, but rather as a state of suffering associated with an extreme state of love, whether for the human beloved or for God, although this may also be a state associated with loss, failure or grief.

Perhaps the greatest medieval literary representations of the loss of the rational self portray individuals possessed by love-malady or love-madness.[30] This idea of lovesickness was prevalent throughout the Middle Ages and Renaissance, and was to recur in notions of hysteria up to the twentieth century. Love was commonly depicted as a force like illness, striking unexpectedly from outside and often represented as a wound caused by the God of Love's arrow. Only the lady could cure this wound, and secular poetry repeatedly employs the image of the lady as physician: in Chaucer's 'A Complaint to His Lady', for instance, she withholds healing from the sick lover, 'The more I love, the more she doth me smerte (hurt), / Thourgh which I see withoute remedye / That from the deeth I may no wyse asterte (escape)' (20–22). Once love had struck, it was depicted as a malady with specific symptoms typical of melancholy: sighing, weeping, swooning, pallor, loss of appetite, weakness and ulti-mately death. In Chaucer's *Troilus and Criseyde*, Troilus manifests these symptoms to an extreme degree, and Chaucer plays on the notion of Troilus as struck by the arrows of the God of Love with sudden and extreme passion for Criseyde, 'that sodeynly hym thoughte he felte dyen, / Right with hire look, the spirit in his herte' (I, 306–7); he feels 'swich wo / That he was wel neigh wood (mad)' (I, 498–99).[31] The symptoms of the extreme melancholy of love also, however, include heightened creativ-ity: love provokes malady and madness, but also the composition of poetry. Chaucer insets Troilus' lyrics, one of which is the first translation of a Petrarch sonnet into English, his hymn to Love, his formal com-plaints, his prayers, and the lovers' *aubades*, as well as their letters. For Troilus, however, melancholy will become destructive rather than life-enhancing. On losing his beloved Criseyde, he is so weakened as to be unrecognisable:

He ne et ne drank, for his malencolye,
And ek from every compaignye he fledde;
This was the lif that al the tyme he ledde.

He so defet* was, that no manere man	*enfeebled
Unneth* hym myghte knowen ther he wente;	*scarcely
So was he lene, and therto pale and wan,	
And feble, that he walketh by potente.*	*crutch (V, 1216–22)

His complaint is of pain around his heart.

In other works, denial or disappointment in love can lead to more extreme forms of madness, which might be classified as mania rather than melancholy. Like Nebuchadnezzar, such grief-stricken lovers lose all rational control, fleeing human civilisation to run wild in the savage outside world. Again this notion is rooted in the theory of the humours, according to which severe emotional distress would produce an excess of one humour, and hence, physiological and mental imbalance. Shakespeare's *Othello* explores this motif with great intensity in the portrayal of Othello's jealous passion, which is echoed by that of Leontes in the *Winter's Tale*, while *King Lear* portrays madness resulting from a different kind of loss in love, in Lear's betrayal by his daughters; the comedies offer us the more light-hearted side of the 'midsummer madness' of love. In medieval romance, from which Shakespeare partly took his cue, love takes the hero into a world of heightened emotional experience, so intense that he may lose all control of his reason, for, as Chrétien de Troyes wrote in the twelfth century, love and reason are always at war, 'Reason ... does not follow Love's command'.[32] The irrationality born of great love can inspire the greatest chivalric achievements: deeds of prowess in war or single combat, or the single-handed undertaking of great adventure. Chrétien's romance of *Le Chevalier de la Charrete* (*The Knight of the Cart*) offers an emblematic instance in the episode of the Sword Bridge: urged on by love for Guinevere, Lancelot takes the most direct but also most dangerous path to rescue her from her abductor, a path that culminates in black, treacherous water crossed only by 'a sharp and gleaming sword', with two lions at its end.[33] Lancelot crosses, much wounded, but guided and healed by love, only to discover that the lions were illusory. Here, as so often in romance, love-madness not reason underpins the greatest adventures.

As well as inspiring great deeds, such extreme passion may overthrow the wits in more incapacitating ways. It is striking that a number of the great Arthurian knights, including Lancelot, Tristan and Yvain, run mad when refused by their ladies, an extreme response to emotion that in medieval romance writing seems to indicate the highest nobility. Thus Chrétien in his *Le Chevalier au Lion* (*The Knight of the Lion*) tells of the knight Yvain, who is so busy gaining honour in tournaments and jousts that he forgets to return to his lady on the appointed day. When he learns that he has lost her love, grief and guilt overthrow his mind:

> Then such a great tempest arose in his head that he went mad; he ripped and tore at his clothing and fled across the fields and plains, leaving his people puzzled and with no idea of where he could be.... afterwards he did not remember anything he had done.

Chrétien recounts how, stealing a bow and arrows, Yvain 'stalked wild animals in the forest and killed them and ate their raw flesh. He lived in the forest like a madman and a savage...'.[34] A hermit takes pity on the naked man, but he is only healed by a precious magical ointment obtained from Morgan le Fay, rubbed on so vigorously by an attentive damsel 'that she expelled the madness and melancholy from his brain'.[35] The scene demonstrates well the notion of madness as descent into a savage or bestial state: it exemplifies the anthropologist Levi-Strauss's distinction between the raw and the cooked, the savage and the civilised, for Yvain, mad, eats the animals' raw flesh. The episode shows clearly the link between madness and guilt, as Yvain atones for his failure in love. Yet it points too to his innate nobility, for even in madness he brings the beasts he catches to feed the hermit. The state of madness marks Yvain's transition to mature, responsible lover: after this, he is able to embark on the series of adventures that will regain his lady and fulfil his own noble nature.

It is striking that in Malory's *Morte Darthur*, written in the fifteenth century but finding its sources in thirteenth-century French prose romance, both Launcelot and Tristram run mad in manners very similar to that of Yvain, Launcelot when Guinevere rejects him, Tristram on believing that La Beale Isode has betrayed him. In both cases, madness marks noble passion and vulnerability. Tristram runs out into the forest, 'and then was he naked and waxed lean and poor of flesh'; he is treated as a madman by the shepherds who feed him, 'And when he did any shrewd deed they would beat him with rods; and so they clipped him with shears and made him like a fool'.[36] Even in his madness, however, he saves the knight Dinant from the 'grimly giant Sir Tauleas' (IX, 20, 215). Launcelot first swoons and then leaps from a window into a garden, 'and there with thorns he was all to-scratched of his visage and his body. And so he ran forth he knew not whither, and was as wild as ever was man; and so he ran two years, and never man had grace to know him' (XI, 8, 288). Yet he too retains his noble instincts: he breaks his chains in the castle where he is cared for in order to take the part of Sir Bliant, when he sees from a window Bliant losing a battle against two knights. These scenes are striking in their use of disjunctive images of violent and complete madness: the greatest of knights are shockingly transformed, losing their reason to run wild in the savage outside world. In both cases, as in that of Yvain, madness proves great passion, and hence great nobility; it is the other side of being the great lover. Natural medicine is no cure for such madness. Tristram is healed by seeing his beloved; Launcelot cannot be cured even by a hermit, but, 'more wooder than he was aforetime' (XII, 3, 296) for lack of food, is attacked by young men as a fool as he runs through the streets of Corbin. The description provides a chilling image of how the mad were treated, 'then all the young men of that city ran after Sir Lancelot, and there they threw turfs at him and gave him many sad strokes' (XII, 3, 296); he can only finally be healed by the Holy Grail itself. Madness proves humanity, vulnerability, depth of passion; the lover is proved precisely by his lack of reason. But we are also made aware of the need for marvellous, magical or divine intervention to cure madness: the return of the beloved, the magical ointment, the Holy Grail, but not a doctor's medicine.

It is not only men who suffer madness. One of the most memorable depictions of a mind overturned in medieval writing occurs in the depiction of Queen Heurodis in the late thirteenth- or early fourteenth-century romance *Sir Orfeo*, a rewriting of the Orpheus and Eurydice story. Orpheus has become an English king; his wife, Heurodis, is abducted by the King of Faery; and after an extraordinary account of Orfeo's journey into the sinister world of Faery, peopled with the bodies of those taken in violent death, and his defeat of the King through the power of his harping, the romance is given a happy ending. It treats the deepest of human fears, that of sudden loss and death, in the eerie narrative of how Heurodis, sleeping under a grafted tree in her orchard, wakes to reveal that she has encountered the King of Faery, who will take her against her will into his land. The violence of Heurodis' vision is manifest in her state of madness and self-mutilation on waking:

> Ac as sone as she gan awake,
> She crid and lothly bere* gan make;   *cry
> She froted* hir honden and hir feet   *scratched
> And crached hir visage – it bled wete.
> Hir riche robe hie all to-rett*   *tore to pieces
> And was reveysed* out of hir wit.[37]   *driven

Despite the guard of a thousand armed knights, she disappears. Heurodis' violent madness is the result not of disappointed desire but of the related passions of loss and grief: she will be taken from her beloved and from the human world. The scene finds a parallel in Shakespeare's portrayal of Ophelia's madness, in which the experience of loss again overturns the mind and results in violence against the self. Once again, madness proves the extremity of passion – of loss, grief, love and suffering.

The response of Orfeo on losing his queen is to adopt the guise of madness: he announces his decision to leave the court and live as a wild man in the woods. His self-imposed exile and wildness function rather as penitential madness might, for they lead him to a state of grace and renewal: in the forest, he will see the Faery Hunt that leads him to the otherworld, where he regains Heurodis. Madness has become a literary topos or motif, so familiar as the emblem of great love that it may be adopted as a self-conscious pose. In the lyric 'I must go walke the woed so wylde', the narrator sees the woods as the appropriate place for his own 'woodnesse' or madness, and Shakespeare plays on the same notion in *A Midsummer Night's Dream*, with the line 'here am I, and wood within this wood', and in *As You Like It* with Orlando's comic love frenzy in the Forest of Arden.[38] Madness, then, could figure in positive ways, not exclusively as the mark of sin, but as the sign of great and noble passion or suffering. It might, as in the cases of Troilus, Lancelot and Tristram, mark a kind of love ecstasy, the kind of emotion so compellingly evoked in Wagner's *Tristan und Isolde*: love, illness, madness, death form a kind of nexus in romance writing, though love-madness does not inevitably signal tragedy.

The ecstatic state was not, however, always occasioned by romantic or secular love. Perhaps most striking of all are the visions of the medieval mystics, often difficult to distinguish from madness even by those who experienced them. For the religious, illness more generally was an important part of experience, viewed as a test sent by God, but also as a special, privileged state. The book of Job asserted the divine source of both illness and healing, and hence the beneficial aspect of illness: 'Behold, happy is the man whom God correcteth: therefore despise not thou the chastening of the Almighty: For he maketh sore, and bindeth up: he woundeth and his hands make whole' (Job 5: 17–18).[39] The New Testament made explicit God's healing power in Christ's miraculous ability to cure the sick, and even to raise the dead; the process of illness and healing was a paradigm too for the promise of forgiveness and immortality brought to sinful man by Christ, the great Physician. The Bible also, however, offered repeated depictions of a visionary or prophetic state something akin to madness, from the visions and prophecies of the Old Testament to the epiphany of Saint Paul on the road to Damascus to John of Patmos's luminously surreal account of the apocalypse and the New Jerusalem in the Book of Revelation. The new emphasis on mysticism in the later Middle Ages produced a new wave of visionary writing. Mysticism responded to what could be seen as a desiccated scholastic tradition by emphasising the individual human relation with Christ and the piety born of emotion. It depended on the affective, the power of images, visual or literary, of Christ and especially of the Passion to move the individual to a new state of religious experience and enlightenment, at its most extreme a state of religious ecstasy or vision. For women who were unlikely to have access to Latin and to the learned theological writings of the Church, this tradition of affective piety was especially formative: the medieval period produced such female mystics as Hildegarde of Bingen, Angela of Foligno, Catherine of Siena, Bridget of Sweden, and in England, Julian of Norwich and Margery Kempe. Mystical vision rewrote, in a sense, the mad frenzy of the rhapsode: it too was a bodily as well as a mental experience, to which the whole being was given over. Visionary experience was encouraged through harsh physical practices: Caroline Walker Bynum, in *Holy Feast and Holy Fast*, explores the possibility that the ascetic monastic life, and particularly deprivation of food, led to a kind of visionary anorexia.[40] Illness provided one way into knowledge of the divine: not only as a welcome test of body and spirit through physical suffering, but also as an altered or detached, privileged state, which could open the soul to vision. Extreme asceticism was a means of achieving a similar state of spiritual otherness through bodily suffering. Julian of Norwich's mystical treatise, *Revelations of Divine Love*, offers a striking instance of the interconnection of illness and vision. She tells how she prayed to experience three miracles, one of which was to approach death in illness:

> In this sikenesse I desired to have all manier peynes bodily and ghostly that I should have if I should dye, with all the dreds and tempests of the fends, except the outpassing of the soule. And this I ment for I would purged be the mercy of God and after lyven more to the worshippe of God because of that sekenesse; and that for the more speede in my deth, for I desired to be soone with my God.[41]

She offers a remarkable description of how, as a result of such an illness in 1373 (at the age of about thirty), she is led to experience her series of visions. Some of these are visually compelling, of Christ withering on the Cross, or the devil taking her by the throat; others are more abstract meditations on different aspects of faith and doctrine; it is in looking back on these visions twenty years later that she writes her *Revelations of Divine Love*. Not only are the visions provoked by illness, however, but also one aspect of Julian's journey of faith is the process of believing that they are not just madness or delirium:

> Than cam a religious person to me and askid me how I ferid. And I seyd I had ravid today, and he leuhe (laughed) loud and inderly (heartily). And I seyd: 'The cross that stod afor my face, methowte it blode fast'. And with this word the person that I spake to waxid al sad and mervelid. (108)

> For on the selfe day that it was shewid, what time that the syte was passid, as a wretch I forsoke it and openly I seid that I had ravid. Than our Lord Iesus of his mercy wold not letten it perish, but he shewid it al agen within, in my soule, with more fulhede (detail), with the blissid lyte of his pretious love, seyand these word full mytyly and full meekly: 'Witt it now wele, it was no raving that thou saw this day....' (113)

Julian evokes too the power of despair in her description of 'the drede of affray (fear) that cummith to a man sodenly' and 'the drede of peyne', and similarly the difficulty of belief, 'doubtfull dread' (118–19): one of her later visions is of two people chattering earnestly yet inaudible and incomprehensible, 'calculated', she says, 'to stirre me to dispeir' (112). For Julian, God's power could be seen in the mysterious and terrifying obscurity of the mind, the failure to understand, as well as in the equally mysterious, marvellous alleviation of this lack of comprehension or vision. Such images of darkness and failure to understand recur across mystical writing: the 'dark night of the soul' of Saint John of the Cross, the Cloud of Unknowing represented by the anonymous Middle English writer, or much later, the darkness of Gerard Manley Hopkins' 'Terrible Sonnets'. For Julian, writing is a means to combat darkness. It is presented as the natural outcome of vision: vision inspires, but also demands to be shown to others. The shift from experience to relation of vision, however, is long: it requires twenty years for Julian's understanding to be clear enough for her to write, and her *Revelations* exist in two versions, indicating her continuing process of contemplation and writing. The placing and probing of ecstatic experience as vision is deeply complex.

In the next generation, Margery Kempe (born c. 1373) offers a rather different model of the process of vision.[42] Margery's *Book* is much more than a mystical text in its dramatic presentation of her life, but also much less of a mystical text in its engagement with theology. Although Margery met Julian of Norwich on her travels, they could scarcely have been more different. Margery was rooted in bourgeois secular society: she bore her husband fourteen children, and was actively involved in business enterprises, attempting both to run a brewing business and to operate a horse-mill. Her book is in some ways a negotiation between secular and spiritual life. Like Julian, however, Margery begins by describing the unpredictability of illness and the divine origin of both illness and healing: 'And than sche toke hir chawmbre and ete alone vi wokys, unto the tyme that owyr Lord mad hir so seke that sche wend to a be ded, and sythen sodeynly he mad hir hool ayen'.[43] Illness triggers Margery's conversion to a holy life: she describes how, after giving birth to her first child, she suffered what would now be termed puerperal insanity, 'sche dyspered of hyr lyfe, wenyng sche mygth not levyn' (52), and then, fearing her confessor's reproof, 'went owt of hir mende and was wondyrlye vexid and labowryd wyth spyrityps half yer, viii wekys and odde days' (54). She vividly describes horrifying visions of devils who torment her, her own 'schrewyd' (evil) words and desire for 'wykkydnesse' (54–55), her attempts to commit suicide, and her self-mutilation. She is forcibly restrained until the sudden miraculous appearance of Christ in her sickroom, sitting by her bed, looking at her with love and saying, 'Dowtyr, why hast thou forsakyn me, and I forsoke nevyr the?' (56). Madness for Margery reflects her sinful state of despair and unbelief:

its demonic torments are a punishment. Christ is the great healer, restoring her mental well-being.

Yet as in the case of Julian of Norwich, Margery's visions can be difficult to distinguish from 'raving'. She converses with Christ, Mary and the saints, welcomes Christ as her lover, participates in his birth and that of the Virgin, offers Mary soothing gruel after the Crucifixion, sees the Sacrament fluttering like a dove, hears the Holy Ghost as the sound of a pair of bellows or a robin redbreast, and experiences various other sensory tokens: sweet smells and melodies, and 'many white thyngys flying al abowte hir on every syde, as thykke in a maner as motys in the sunne; it weryn ryth sotyl and comfortabyl, and the brygtare that the sunne schyned, the bettyr sche myth se hem' (192–93). Modern readers have been tempted to interpret Margery's symptoms medically (the specks, for instance, as the ocular disturbance of migraine), but such interpretations are finally unsatisfying: to Margery, such experiences were visionary, inspiring extraordinary actions, but also the writing of the book itself. Although, like Julian, she fears 'illusyons and deceytys' (141) and needs affirmation, Margery's belief in her experiences converts her to a religious life of chastity and asceticism, but also extraordinary action. Her pilgrimages take her as far as the Holy Land, while her radical speaking, especially to Church authorities, causes her to be repeatedly suspected of heresy.

It seems certain from her book, however, that what attracted most attention was Margery's apparently 'mad' behaviour of extreme 'crying'. Abnormal behaviour was typical of the mystic, and there are numerous medieval accounts of the physical manifestations of vision: swoons, convulsions, catalepsy, compulsive weeping and shrieking. Margery repeatedly describes the experience of 'gret wepyng and gret sobbyng', 'that many man and woman also wondryd on hir therfore (209, 208). While tears are very frequently associated with spiritual and visionary experience in mystical writing, Margery's 'cryings' evidently surpass any ordinary weeping. She describes how she first experienced them in Jerusalem:

And sche had so gret compassyon and so gret peyn to se owyr Lordys peyn that sche myt not kepe hirself fro krying and roryng, thow sche schuld a be ded therfor .... And this maner of crying enduryd many yerys aftyr this tyme, for owt that any man myt do, and therfor sufferyd sche mych despyte and mech reprefe. The cryeng was so lowde and so wondyrful that it made pepyl astoynd, les than thei had herd it beforn and er elly[s] that thei knew the cawse of the crying. And sche had hem so oftyntymes that thei madyn hir ryth weyke in hir bodyly myghtys, and namely yf sche herd of owyr Lordys Passyon. (163–64)

Margery describes how the crying might occur anywhere, sometimes only once a month but sometimes fourteen times a day, and how, the more she tried to contain it, the more it would burst out amazingly loudly, to be followed by 'passyng gret swetnesse of devocyon and hey contemplacyon' (165). By no means all Margery's contemporaries were so moved by her cryings: 'many man merveyled ful meche what hir eyled' and 'weryn wroth' (245, 225). In Church, congregations and priests object, for her noise drowns out the service; her fellow pilgrims abandon her or treat her with contempt, 'demyng sche had ben vexyd wyth sum evyl spiryt, er a sodeyn sekenes' (186). She is disarmingly candid about the responses elicited by her behaviour:

> ... summe seyd it was a wikkyd spiryt vexid hir; sum seyd it was a sekenes; sum seyd sche had dronkyn to mech wyn; some bannyd (cursed) hir; sum wisshed sche had ben in the havyn (harbour); sum wolde sche had ben in the se in a bottumles boyt; and so ich man as hym thowte. Other gostly (spiritual) men lovyd hir and favowrd hir the mor. (165)

There is no doubt that the line between madness and vision appeared blurred in the mystical experiences of Margery.

As in the case of Julian's *Revelations*, Margery's writing does not immediately follow her visionary experiences. Rather, her book requires a lengthy gestation period: it is not directly the product of an extreme mental state, but of the recollection of such experience. Twenty years after her first vision, Margery is moved to have her story told as 'a schort tretys and a comfortabyl for synful wrecchys', which would reveal Christ's marvellous works by narrating 'how mercyfully, how benyngly, and how charytefully he meved and stered a synful caytyf unto hys love' (41). Margery herself could neither read nor write, and the book is thus complicated in that its scribes almost certainly edited it as well as copying it. After employing an Englishman living in Germany to write her life, Margery brings the book to a priest who finds it 'so evel wretyn that he cowd lytyl skyll theron (make little sense of it), for it was neithyr good Englysch ne Dewch, ne the lettyr was nat schapyn ne formyd as other letters ben' (47). This man sends her to another priest, who is eventually inspired to be able to read and copy the illegible text, which he dates to 1436. At this late juncture, while the book was being rewritten, Margery added a second book, ten more chapters, which detailed her life since she completed the first book. The book, then, is actually at several removes from its creator and its subject matter: Margery speaks twenty years after the events she describes, her words are copied by one semi-literate scribe, rewritten by a second scribe, and revised at her own direction. No more than Julian's can it be seen as the immediate result of mental disorder, but its origins are rooted in Margery's extreme mental state. The book is most characterised by its extraordinarily lively individual voice, its evocation of personal struggle and inexplicable visionary experience, and it stands as the first autobiography in English.

We may place alongside Julian of Norwich and Margery Kempe one final example, that of the fifteenth-century poet Thomas Hoccleve, a writer who saw himself not as divinely inspired but as seriously mentally ill, but again one whose illness both led eventually to a creative state and provided a subject. Hoccleve's poems include the earliest account in English of the process of recovery from mental illness told from the sufferer's viewpoint. Hoccleve, a civil servant, was a clerk at the Privy Seal, and was, he tells us, encouraged by Chaucer in his writing of poetry: he produced a variety of religious and secular verse, as well as a major poem on the ideal virtues of a ruler, *The Regiment of Princes*. In 1416, Hoccleve succumbed for several months to severe mental illness; although he returned to work, five years passed before he wrote again. His final series of poems comes directly out of his experience of illness and gradual recovery: it comprises the autobiographical *Complaint* and *Dialogue with a Friend*, two moral tales and a poem on mortality. The *Complaint* is a lament on Hoccleve's fall from public favour, a defence of his sanity, and finally a farewell to his sorrow as he considers God's favour in alleviating his sickness and turns to the hope offered by Reason. Its opening is deeply melancholy, as the poet describes autumn, 'the broun sesoun of Mighelmesse', the trees robbed of their leaves, which lie dead and trampled underfoot, and the 'chaunge' in the poet's 'herte roote' as he remembers that 'stablenesse in this world is ther noon; / Ther is no thing / but chaunge and variance': Death will thrust everyone underfoot.[44] Hoccleve then moves to a consideration of his illness of five years before, and his treatment since. He does not offer great detail about his illness, but refers to it as a 'wyldnesse' (107), 'the wylde infirmitee / ... which me out of myself / caste and threew' (40–42); it includes loss of memory, 'the substance / of my memorie / Wente to pleye / as for a certein space' (50–51), and Hoccleve repeatedly uses the image of his wits wandering and returning home. Public records show that he was given a special loan and payment of his annuity at that time, and it seems most likely that he suffered from severe, perhaps manic depression, although it is possible that, as his Friend later suggests, his illness resulted from excessive study, and was what might now be called a nervous breakdown. Hoccleve, however, does not see his illness in these terms, but as caused by a humoural imbalance, restored by God: 'Right so / thogh þat my wit / were a pilgrym / And wente fer from hoom / he cam agayn. / God me voidid / of the greuous venym / Þat had infectid / and wyldid my brayn' (232–35). He seems to envisage an excess of black bile, causing an extreme form of melancholia. Hoccleve describes his subsequent rejection by society in terms still very resonant: people turn their heads away from him in the street, flee, say his sickness will return in time, or 'Whan passynge hete is' (92), and claim that he looks wild and changed, is jumpy and irrational, wandering in his steps and 'al braynseek' (129). His response is silence, 'I had lost my tonges keye' (144); he is 'droupynge and heuy / and al woo bistaad' (146), all symptoms of melancholy, and he writes no poetry for five years.

This is his state of mind when the poem begins: his spirits labour, his heart is changeable, he is sleepless, suffering from the 'thoghtful maladie' (21), and it is this that triggers the writing of the poem. In writing his *Complaint*, Hoccleve may be seen as working through his deep melancholy, in the late stages of his recovery from the severe mental illness that began by casting him from himself. The poem offers a record of his illness, but also a critique of the social condemnation of madness and the general failure to believe in healing, and a defence of Hoccleve's own reason. It shifts in tone from sorrow and anger to the recognition that there is hope for recovery, and that Reason (religious and philosophical argument) can offer a new, more optimistic mode of being, 'now myself / to myself haue ensurid / For no swich wondrynge [of others] aftir this to mourne' (304–5). Hoccleve presents himself as scourged, corrected and healed by God: 'He yaf me wit / and he took it away / Whan þat he sy / þat I it mis despente / And yaf ageyn / whan it was to his pay' (400–2).

The latter part of Hoccleve's poem recalls the emphasis of Julian and Margery, as he turns to admiration for God as the great Physician, with the power to alleviate illness as swiftly as He caused it, 'If þat a leche / curid had me so – / As they lakke alle / þat science and might – / A name he sholde / han had for euere mo / What cure he had doon / to so seek a wight, / And yit my purs / he wolde han maad ful light; / But Ihesu / of his grace pacient, / Axith nat / but of gilt amendement' (85–91). The lines are poignant, for they speak of the impossibility of human doctors providing a cure for mental illness, and of the complete and sudden enigma of such illness, which is seen as 'the strook of God' (79). Hoccleve's way of coming to terms with his illness is to place it as a chastisement but also a blessing from God, in opening out his understanding of divine providence and the possibility of grace, for, he says, 'he in me / hath shewid his miracle' (95).

For Hoccleve, then, madness is both subject and inspiration. His writing of the poem stems from both aspects of madness: he looks back on the horrifying experience of wild infirmity, of being cast out of the self, but also looks to a new state of enlightenment, the process of repentance and hope, which the miracle of healing has triggered. This is the creative state of heightened experience and intensity of feeling, 'the thoghtful maladie' following complete disorder of the mind, and it is then that Hoccleve's poem, like the visions of Margery and Julian, is written. It is not complete madness, the state of being wholly outside the self, that allows for the creative act of writing, but the slow process of emergence from that state of otherness, when the 'lyric glow' of illness is still felt, but the rational self is in control of picking up the pen and writing.

It is here that the real anguish of mental illness connects with the literary traditions of madness as penitential process and manifestation of extreme love, and with the divinely inspired madness of mystical vision. In each case the experience of having been cast out of the self may lead, ultimately, to a state of realisation, fulfilment, or vision, to show the possibility of grace. Yet such a state occurs only after the experience of extreme mental disorder, in recovery or contemplation – and only for some. Romantic creativity is not situated in the agony of madness itself, as Hoccleve shows so clearly, but in the transitional state between illness and recovery, or between madness and rationality, for those who are fortunate enough to experience that transition, and to find inspiration within it.

Notes

1 Shoshana Felman, *Writing and Madness (Literature/Philosophy/Psychoanalysis)*, trans. Martha Noel Evans et al. (Palo Alto, 2003), p. 19.
2 Pindar, *The Pythian Odes*, in *Pindar's Victory Songs*, trans. Frank J. Nisetich (Baltimore, 1980), Pythian 5, turn 3, p. 192, cited by Raymond A. Anselment, *The Realms of Apollo: Literature and Healing in Seventeenth-Century England* (Newark and London, 1995), p. 11. Apollo was also the patron of the Pythian games, which Pindar celebrates here.
3 Plato, *Ion; or, of the Iliad*, trans. Percy Bysshe Shelley, in *Five Dialogues of Plato*, ed. A. D. Lindsay, Everyman's Library (London, 1938), pp. 1–16 (pp. 6–7).
4 Plato, *Phaedrus*, in *Phaedrus and the Seventh and Eighth Letters*, trans. Walter Hamilton (Harmondsworth, 1973) pp. 19–103 (p. 48).
5 Plato, *Timaeus*, in *Timaeus and Critias*, trans. Desmond Lee (Harmondsworth, 1971) pp. 27–126 (p. 99).
6 Plato, *Plato's 'The Republic'*, trans. G. M. A. Grube (Indianapolis, 1982), Book X, p. 249; see also Plato's discussion of poets in Books II and III. Frederick Burwick discusses Plato's attitudes to poetry and madness in *Poetic Madness and the Romantic Imagination* (University Park, PA, 1996), in particular pp. 21–22. See also Robin Downie's essay in this volume, pp. 48–62.
7 Michel Foucault, *Madness and Civilization: A History of Insanity in the Age of Reason*, trans. R. Howard (London, 1967, repr. 1989), p. 537. Originally published as *Folie et déraison: histoire de la folie à l'âge classique*, Civilisations d'hier et d'aujourd'hui (Paris, 1961). Felman cites this phrase, p. 52.
8 See Roy Porter, *Madness: A Brief History* (Oxford, 2002), pp. 92–100.
9 For discussion of attitudes to, and theories and treatment of, madness in the medieval period, see in particular Penelope B. R. Doob, *Nebuchadnezzar's Children: Conventions of Madness in Middle English Literature* (New Haven, CT, 1974), pp. 1–53, and Simon Kemp, *Medieval Psychology*, Contributions in Psychology 14 (New York, 1990), pp. 111–33. See also Roy Porter's account in *The Greatest Benefit to Mankind: A Medical History of Humanity from Antiquity to the Present* (London, 1997), pp. 127–28 and in *Madness: A Brief History*, pp. 89–92. Other studies of madness in the medieval period include: Basil Clarke, *Mental Disorder in Earlier Britain* (Cardiff, 1975); Stanley W. Jackson, 'Unusual Medical States in Medieval Europe: I, Medical Syndromes of Mental Disorder: 400–1100 A.D.', *Journal of the History of Medicine and Allied Sciences* 27 (1972), pp. 262–97; Richard Neugebauer, 'Treatment of the Mentally Ill in Medieval and Early Modern England: A Reappraisal', *Journal of the History of the Behavioural Sciences* 14 (1978) and, 'Medieval and Early Modern Theories of Mental Illness', *Archives of General Psychiatry* 36 (1979), pp. 477–83; and C. H. Talbot, *Medicine in Medieval*

England (London, 1967). The following discussion is particularly indebted to that of Kemp.

10   See Kemp's refutation of these myths, pp. 112–14.

11   Julius Zupitza, ed., *Bischofs Wærferth von Worcester Übersetzung der Dialoge Gregors des Grossen*, Bibliothek der Angelsächsischen Prosa 5 (Leipzig, 1900), Bk 1, ix, pp. 30–31.

12   Kemp, p. 136.

13   See Porter's summary, *The Greatest Benefit to Mankind*, p. 9.

14   See Kemp's full discussion, pp. 117–21, and Doob's examination of the causes of madness, pp. 19–30.

15   Kemp, p. 118.

16   Geoffrey Chaucer, *The Knight's Tale*, in *The Riverside Chaucer*, 3rd edn, ed. Larry D. Benson (Oxford, 1987), lines 1374–76; this passage is cited by Kemp, p. 119. All subsequent references to Chaucer's works will be from this edition and will be cited by line number.

17   See Kemp's discussion, pp. 121–25, and Doob, pp. 36–45.

18   See Kemp, p. 124.

19   See Kemp's discussion, pp. 125–28.

20   Bracton, *Bracton de legibus et consuetudinibus Angliae: Bracton on the Laws and Customs of England*, ed. George E. Woodbine, trans. Samuel E. Thorne, 4 vols (Cambridge, MA, in ass. with Selden Society, 1968–77), vol. 2, p. 424, cited by Kemp, p. 126.

21   Kemp, p. 126.

22   Kemp, p. 127.

23   See Kemp, p. 128.

24   Kemp, p. 151.

25   Doob, p. 8 and see her discussion of the relation of the Fall to madness, pp. 7–10.

26   Kemp, p. 115.

27   R. F. Yeager, *John Gower's Poetic: The Search For A New Arion*, Publications of the John Gower Society 2 (Cambridge, 1990) pp. 153–154. See John Gower, *Confessio Amantis*, in *The English Works of John Gower*, ed. G. C. Macaulay, 2 vols, Early English Text Society ES 81 and 82 (Oxford, 1900) Book V, line 5627. All subsequent references to *Gower's Confessio Amantis* will be from this edition and will be cited by book and line number.

28   Doob offers a detailed analysis of Nebuchadnezzar's madness, pp. 54–94 (for her discussion of Gower, see pp. 86–90).

29   Robert Burton, *The Anatomy of Melancholy*, ed. Floyd Dell and Paul Jordan-Smith (New York, 1951) Part I, Section 1, Member 1, Subsection 1, pp. 118–19; the second passage is cited and discussed by Doob, p. 10.

30   For a comprehensive discussion, see Mary Frances Wack, *Lovesickness in the Middle Ages: The 'Viaticum' and its Commentaries*, Middle Ages Series (Philadelphia, 1990).

31   For an excellent introduction to *Troilus*, see Barry Windeatt, *Troilus and Crisyede*, Oxford Guides to Chaucer (Oxford, 1992), especially pp. 234–40, on 'Sickness and Death'.

32   Chrétien de Troyes, *The Knight of the Cart (Lancelot)*, in *Arthurian Romances*, trans. William W. Kibler (Harmondsworth, 1991) pp. 207–94 (p. 212).

33   Chrétien de Troyes, *The Knight of the Cart*, p. 244.

34   Chrétien de Troyes, *The Knight with the Lion (Yvain)*, in *Arthurian Romances*, pp. 295–380 (p. 330).

35 Chrétien de Troyes, *The Knight with the Lion*, pp. 332–33.
36 Sir Thomas Malory, *Le Morte Darthur: The Winchester Manuscript*, ed. Helen Cooper, Oxford World's Classics (Oxford, 1998), IX, 18, p. 214. All subsequent references to Malory's *Morte Darthur* will be from this edition, and will be cited by Caxton's book and chapter numbers, and page number (I use this slightly abridged version as the most accessible edition of the manuscript).
37 *Sir Orfeo*, in *Middle English Verse Romances*, ed. Donald B. Sands, Exeter Medieval English Texts and Studies (Exeter, 1986), pp 185–200 (p. 188, lines 53–58).
38 See *Secular Lyrics of the XIVth and XVth Centuries*, ed. Rossell Hope Robbins, 2nd edn (Oxford, 1955), no. 20, and *A Midsummer Night's Dream* II, I, 192.
39 See in particular Anselment's discussion of the divine origins of illness, pp. 25–30.
40 Caroline Walker Bynum, *Holy Feast and Holy Fast: The Religious Significance of Food to Medieval Women* (Berkeley, 1987).
41 Julian of Norwich, *A Revelation of Love*, ed. Marion Glasscoe, revised edn, Exeter Medieval English Texts and Studies (Exeter, 1993), p. 3. All subsequent references to Julian's *Revelations* will be from this edition and will be cited by page number.
42 Roy Porter offers a detailed discussion of Margery Kempe's life and autobiography as 'an account of a woman going mad', but also exercising control over her destiny, *A Social History of Madness: Stories of the Insane* (London, 1987, 1996), pp. 103–12.
43 Margery Kempe, *The Book of Margery Kempe*, ed. Barry Windeatt, Longman Annotated Texts (London, 2000, reprinted Cambridge, 2004), p. 158. All subsequent references to Margery's *Book* will be from this edition and will be cited by page number.
44 Thomas Hoccleve, *Thomas Hoccleve's Complaint and Dialogue*, ed. J. A. Burrow, Early English Text Society 313 (Oxford, 1999), lines, 2, 7, 9–10. All subsequent references to Hoccleve's *Complaint* will be to this edition, using the edited text, and will be cited by line number.

5

'Inexpressibly Dreadful': Depression, Confession and Language in Eighteenth-Century Britain

Allan Ingram

In 1691, at the age of thirty-three, Timothy Rogers, by then a Nonconformist minister in Berkshire, published his *Discourse Concerning Trouble of Mind*. It was dedicated to his patron, Lady Mary Lane, to whom Rogers addresses a long 'Epistle Dedicatory': 'To the very much HONOURED and RESPECTED LADY, The Lady Mary Lane'. Apart from confirming the encouragement, advice and understanding she has given him, Rogers also gives Lady Mary the most heartfelt admiration. 'You have never', he says,

> been afflicted with that Distemper and those Anxieties of Soul whereof I treat in the following Book, and I heartily pray you never may: For MELANCHOLLY is the worst of all Distempers; and those sinking and guilty Fears which it brings along with it, are inexpressibly dreadful.[1]

Not that Lady Mary has not had cause for depression, having 'been in manifold Afflictions' and had 'several very great Losses':

> You lost some years ago a Father, who was indeed, in all respects ... worthy to be loved.... You lost a Mother, whom all that knew her greatly valued.... And not to mention other Losses, you have lost several Children, in whom there was all the sweetness of youth, all that good temper, and those blooming appearances of hopefulness which could make such little Plants desirable.[2]

However, she has 'born even so great a Loss with a submissive and a Christian Patience, as knowing that you have not so much cause to mourn for those that are gone as to rejoyce in those that are left; and who are a very great Comfort to you; and may they long be so'.[3]

'Inexpressibly dreadful.' Here is the subject of this paper, the expression of depression, the acknowledgement of it, even the confession of it, its paradoxes, its dilemmas, in writing by three people between the 1680s and the latter part of the eighteenth century. Two are women: Hannah Allen, a little-known young Nonconformist widow from Derbyshire, who published her account of her depressive breakdown in 1683, and Anne Finch, Countess of Winchilsea, whose poetry has been printed and read since she first began to publish in 1701. How did these two women, in their different ways and in their respective written forms, express, unlike patient Lady Mary Lane, their trouble of mind? In contrast, however, both in terms of gender and literary form, I begin with a man, one from later in the eighteenth century, quite a well-known one, a life-long depressive and articulator of his depression in journal and letter, James Boswell.

Boswell was a compulsive recorder. 'For my own part', he wrote in 1783, 'I have so long accustomed myself to write a Diary, that when I omit it the day seems to be lost, though for the most part I put down nothing but immaterial facts which it can serve no purpose of any value to record'.[4] He first began to keep a journal in 1758, when he was seventeen, and from 1762 until his death in 1795 he maintained, more or less consistently, the habit of writing up, often in minute detail, and often after a delay of days or even weeks, the events, thoughts, conversations and transactions of his life. 'I should live', he observes in his journal during an optimistic period in his mid thirties, 'no more than I can record, as one should not have more corn growing than one can get in. There is a waste of good if it be not preserved.'[5] Over a lifetime, naturally, there is great variety in the mood and materials that are gathered into Boswell's journal, but two features persist, often in alternating relation to each other: his exuberance, and his depression. For Boswell was also a hypochondriac.

Hypochondria, melancholy, depression pervaded every aspect of Boswell's life and of his writing, manifesting themselves as a sense of personal worthlessness, as excruciating guilt for things done, or not done, or simply as an undeniable awareness of the futility of human existence, often accompanied by religious doubts. As he writes to his friend John Johnston from Holland in 1764, 'I saw all things as so precarious and vain that I had no relish of them, no views to fill my mind, no motive to incite me to action.... Black melancholy again took dominion over me.'[6] Moreover, as the existence of this letter indicates, Boswell also felt the overwhelming urge to tell others of his depression. That which, in Rogers' words, was 'inexpressibly dreadful' nevertheless, in Boswell as much as Rogers and, as we shall see, in Hannah Allen and Anne Finch, demanded to be told and retold in a lifetime of barely adequate phrases. Certainly, as Philip Martin has put it, 'his extensive reflections on it in essays, letters, and journals did little to improve his condition'.[7] But what was more potentially disastrous was that for Boswell the expressive urge was an instinct that, he feared, also laid him perpetually open to ridicule or to censure. In London, in 1786, for example, he talks of his low spirits to his fellow bar counsel, adding in his journal account: 'This was imprudent. But mental pain could not be endured quietly.'[8] Boswell never endured mental pain quietly, but he did find ways of sharing it that reduced the risk of ridicule. He talked with and exchanged letters with friends, especially those of a hypochondriac tendency – with John Johnston; with Bennet Langton, with whom he agreed on the 'deceitfulness of all our hopes of enjoyment on earth'; or with Andrew Erskine: 'On comparing notes, I found he differed from me in this: that he at no time had any ambition or the least inclination to distinguish himself in active life, having a perpetual consciousness or imagination that he could not go through with it.'[9] The need for such safe intimacy was also a motive behind his writing a series of essays, published as *The Hypochondriack* in the *London Magazine* between 1777 and 1783, a series in which Boswell, writing anonymously, offered advice and distraction to fellow sufferers. But the main means whereby he confessed the forms and frequency of his hypochondria, and thereby reined in what he refers to as 'a kind of strange feeling as if I wished nothing to be secret that concerns myself', was in the privacy, or the comparative privacy, of his journal.[10]

The compulsion to tell, for Boswell, covered a range of activities and needs apart from his recurring depression. Some of these, inevitably, also had the tendency to feed that depression. They are also, of course, characteristic of the freedom of movement and morals available to an upper middle-class male lawyer that was not available to a Derbyshire widow, a dependent Nonconformist minister, or even to a depressed countess. I refer in particular to Boswell's frequent marital infidelities, when his behaviour is written up sometimes with relish, sometimes with regret, and often with a mixture of both. What is interesting, though, is the fact that he wrote it up at all, the apparent psychological function that writing served, and its relation to his depression, especially when, as often seemed to happen, his wife Margaret found and read his journal. A sequence of events that took place in Edinburgh between November and December 1776 is illustrative of this relation between action and depression in Boswell's temperament, and within the journal he was living as he wrote it, between the language of re-creation and the language of depressive reflection, for they are mutually and intimately dependent. On Monday 25 November, Boswell, who should have been working at law-papers, instead argues with Margaret, and leaves the house. Later, 'coming home at five,' he writes, 'I met a young slender slut with a red cloak in the street and went with her to Barefoots Parks and madly ventured coition. It was', he adds, 'a short and almost insensible gratification of lewdness. I was vexed to think of it.'[11] Vexed or not, two evenings later, in the High Street, he 'met a plump hussy who called herself Peggy Grant' and 'went with her to a field behind the Register Office, and boldly lay with her. This was desperate risking.' It was, Boswell interjects, 'one of the coldest nights I ever remember'. Even more 'desperate' information is revealed in the following day's entry:

The girl with whom I was last night had told me she lodged in Stevenlaw's Close, and at my desire engaged to be at the head of it generally at eight in the evening, in case I should be coming past. I thought I could not be in more danger of disease by one more enjoyment the very next evening, so went tonight; but she was not there.

He finishes the day by observing: 'I was shocked that the father of a family should go amongst strumpets; but there was rather an insensibility about me to virtue, I was so sensual. Perhaps I should not write all this' – 'all this', from Monday through till Thursday, in fact being written on Friday 29 November. On Sunday 1 December, however, a crisis is reached. First of all, Boswell, at church listening to a sermon, is already sketching out his evening:

I must *confess* that I planned, even when sober, that I would in the evening try to find Peggy Grant, and, as I had risked with her, take a full enjoyment.... About eight I got into the street and made Cameron, the chairman, inquire for Peggy Grant.... He brought her out, and I took her to the New Town, and in a mason's shed in St. Andrew's Square lay with her twice.

Later, at home and sober, but 'in a confused, feverish frame', Boswell finds his wife suspicious: 'My dear wife asked me if I had not been about mischief. I at once confessed it. She was very uneasy, and I was ashamed and vexed at my licentiousness. Yet', adds Boswell, ending the day's entry (written the following day, Monday 2 December), 'my conscience was not alarmed; so much had I accustomed my mind to think such indulgence permitted.' Telling, for Boswell, was clearly an important dimension of living, as if the actual experience remained incomplete for him until it had also been re-created in writing, within the confessional of his journal. The prose is energetic, active, with an eye for the memorable detail – the 'young slender slut with a red cloak'. It revives and re-enacts as it goes. And yet it does not simply re-create, for Boswell is also his own moral commentator, his own confessor: 'I was vexed to think of it'; 'This was desperate risking'; and especially 'Perhaps I should not write all this.' There is a mixing of time scales, with Boswell the writer, the man of words, the confessing voice, looking back on Boswell the actor, the misbehaver, the confessed for, so that the journal reality emerges as a superior, more roundedly truthful reality than a life simply lived with no account kept. Lived reality became, apparently, more real by virtue of giving itself over to language, of conceding its deeds, thoughts, layers, timescales to the written word, of making a perpetual confession of itself.

On this occasion, Boswell's confession to his wife of his mischief – and again the event is illustrative – was not the end of the matter. The actual confession to Margaret is, of course, itself confessed within the journal, and therefore forms part of the more truthful reality of Boswell's privately known self. One week later, on Sunday 8 December, Mrs Boswell 'insisted to read this my journal,' and,

> finding in it such explicit instances of licentiousness, she was much affected and told me that she had come to a resolution never again to consider herself as my *wife*; though for the sake of her children and mine, as a *friend*, she would preserve appearances. When I saw her in great uneasiness, and dreaded somewhat – though not with much apprehension – her resolution, I was awakened from my dream of licentiousness, and saw my bad conduct in a shocking light. I was really agitated, and in a degree of despair.... At night I calmly meditated to reform.[12]

In one sense, the two realities have abruptly been brought together, and the private, more truthful reality has been forced to acknowledge itself within the real lived world. It has been exposed for the sham thing it is, a confession with no comeback, no penances, no risk. Boswell is forced to see his conduct, his mental prevarications, his moral shiftiness, as cheap, self-serving and hurtful: as 'inexpressibly dreadful'. He is genuinely moved, sufficiently moved to write up the whole week, from Tuesday till Sunday, on the very evening of the calamity.

In another sense, however, the journal is reinforced as the superior reality, and this happens in two ways. Firstly, Margaret Boswell's reading actually turns Boswell's journal into a yet more genuine confession – more genuinely a confession than Boswell intended when he wrote it – and a still more roundedly true confession. Not only does she find out the whole truth, but her reading is also an endorsement, a consummation of one of the deepest instincts behind Boswell's writing, the 'strange feeling' to have 'nothing to be secret that concerns myself'. She is a third party who brings an outside eye to the confessing voice, the confessed actor, and thereby reintegrates it into the reality of deeds, feelings, people, out from the world of language in which it has been privileged to exist. And she is the woman for whose stay-at-home eye this free-roving reporter has acted, erred, reflected, confessed and grown miserable.

But secondly, and inevitably, the journalist goes on. Language can never be outflanked by life. Boswell writes up five days in order to get to the sixth, Sunday 8 December, and to record the catastrophe, to confess his 'despair', after which he leaves off writing for another week. The brutal enforcement into the world of Mrs Boswell, the children, appearances, the making of the journal a genuine confessional, is itself in its turn confessed, reincorporated into the more roundedly truthful linguistic reality, even more roundedly truthful, in fact, since the endorsement by Margaret and the outside eye.

Not that Boswell existed easily between these realities. There is, indeed, in his writing a constant ambiguity, a series of tensions between the self that acted and the self that was conscious of having participated in action. The reflective self can reflect at times with satisfaction on the self that has acted, as upon his arrival in London in 1762:

> Since I came up, I have begun to acquire a composed genteel character very different from a rattling uncultivated one which for some time past I have been fond of. I have discovered that we may be in some degree whatever character we choose.[13]

The reflective self can even reflect with satisfaction on its existence within the reflective medium, on its own facility with language:

> How easily and cleverly do I write just now! I am really pleased with myself; words come skipping to me like lambs upon Moffat Hill; and I turn my periods smoothly and imperceptibly like a skilful wheelwright turning tops in a turning-loom.[14]

But more often the reflective self is forced to respond with distress, shame, censure at what it is obliged to record. So, in Scotland in March 1777, he 'drank outrageously at Whitburn and at Livingstone and at some low ale-house, and arrived at Edinburgh very drunk. It was shocking in me to come home to my dear wife in such a state.'[15] Or in London in March 1776 he finds my 'moral principle as to chastity was absolutely eclipsed.... I was in the miserable state of those whom the apostle represents as working all uncleanness with greediness.... This is an exact state of my mind at the time. It shocks me to review it.'[16] Even in the generally buoyant record that is the London Journal, Boswell has to observe: 'I now see the sickly suggestions of inconsistent fancy with regard to the Scotch bar in their proper colours. Good heaven!... I shudder when I think of it. I am vexed at such a distempered suggestion's being inserted in my journal....'[17]

Part of this tension is to do with his desire to preserve 'good' in the journal, to make a genuine harvest of his life. More deep-seated, though, is Boswell's confusion over the relation between two dimensions of reality – between action and reflection, between the world as lived and the world as confessed. Where, in particular, is there any security in identity when the recording self is constantly to be appalled by the active self, is obliged, in fact, to set down actions and moods that would be better, safer, though less truthful, if let go into oblivion? This confusion is particularly acute for the hypochondriac who, as Boswell writes in *The Hypochondriack*, is perpetually in need of reassurance about his own stability:

> Nothing is more disagreeable than for a man to find himself unstable and changeful. An Hypochondriack is very liable to this uneasy imperfection,

in so much that sometimes there remains only a mere consciousness of identity. His inclinations, his tastes, his friendships, even his principles, he with regret feels, or imagines he feels are all shifted, he knows not how. This is owing to a want of firmness of mind.[18]

When there are two realities, for the hypochondriac the question that most acutely demands answering, and which never can be answered, is not which is the more real, but which is the more sane.

These uncertainties make the journalistic confession of hypochondria particularly distressing. Early in his life, Boswell looked optimistically even on this aspect of keeping a journal. Not only will he 'preserve many things that would otherwise be lost in oblivion' but he will 'find daily employment for myself, which will save me from indolence and help to keep off the spleen'.[19] Elsewhere, he speculates as to whether writing might not actually transplant depression from his mind to the page: 'Lord Monboddo said on Saturday that writing down hurt the memory. Could I extract the hypochondria from my mind, and deposit it in my journal, writing down would be very valuable.'[20] More often, though, Boswell resents the constant, and increasingly frequent, presence of depression in his journal, not least because recording, he feels, gives validity to what should not be acknowledged: 'I really believe', he writes from Holland in 1764, 'that these grievous complaints should not be vented; they should be considered as absurd chimeras, whose reality should not be allowed in words.'[21]

The relation between depression and writing is acutely problematic. Hypochondria was a condition that was for Boswell an undeniably real feature of his life, yet to be always recording it was perhaps to offer it an endorsement that it did not deserve. But the urge to tell was itself a powerful factor within the hypochondriac temperament. Moreover, if confession of so major a part of his existence was to be denied, then where was the truth of the journal to be found?

These issues, always underlying Boswell's attitudes towards his journal and its writing, are especially accentuated in the recording of the final years of his life, from the mid 1780s until 1795, following the death of Johnson, Boswell's own move from Scotland to London, and Margaret's death in 1789. Boswell, while working on the *Life of Johnson*, experienced almost unrelieved depression:

> What sunk me very low was the sensation that I was precisely as when in wretched low spirits thirty years ago, without any addition to my character from having had the friendship of Dr. Johnson and many eminent men, made the tour of Europe, and Corsica in particular, and written two very successful Books. I was as a board on which fine figures had been painted, but which some corrosive application had reduced to its original nakedness.[22]

He castigates the journal he is keeping: 'What a wretched Register is this! "A Lazarhouse it seem'd." It is the Journal of a diseased mind.'[23] The mentality that had been in doubt over so many years of recording, held in check or endorsed in words, is revealed for what it is. The ambiguities have cleared: confirmed by the journal, he has a diseased mind.

Boswell's journal writing is so palsied by depression that language itself can scarcely be brought to persist in giving an account of it. Boswell resident in London, for so long the absolute height of his ambitions, is unrelievedly miserable. At last, after weeks of dreariness, he finally makes, in what is virtually a footnote to his journal entry, the confession that in effect concedes defeat. Wednesday 10 October 1787: 'N.B. Understood *not well* till a change is marked.'[24] The moment is crucial. The lifelong battle to keep pace in language with the events of his life, to live no more than he could record, has been lost, not because Boswell has been living too much, but too little. Language, after all, was outflanked by life, the confessor by the confessed, the re-creative energies of the world of language by the inertness, the exhausted capacities of habitual depression.

If Boswell's journal had been a place for confessional re-creation, in all the variety of his life's activities, this defeat has other implications, for confession, especially of the order of Boswell's, depends on language telling more truthfully, in its privileged space, than deeds, actions, appearances can. But language, now, for Boswell, has nothing to tell, or rather what it tells is nothing pertinent to what is really the case. It is appearance that is given over to the language of the journal, while confession is reduced to silence. That which is more roundedly true is to be marked not in language but by the absence of language, 'understood' until 'a change is marked'. Silence, when all is said and done, is conceded to be the appropriate medium for a state of mind that is 'inexpressibly dreadful', and 'whose reality should not be allowed in words'.

Timothy Rogers' book, from which I quoted earlier, has the full title, *A Discourse Concerning Trouble of Mind and the Disease of Mellancholy, In Three Parts. Written for the Use of such as are, or have been Exercised by the same. By Timothy Rogers, M.A. who was long afflicted with both*. Rogers clearly, in the passages with which I began, is citing Lady Mary Lane as a model of proper patience, of mild acceptance of heaven's decrees, and of Christian goodness through the course of a lifetime's afflictions, in contrast to himself and to those about to be addressed in his book. He is also, though perhaps less advertently, indicating thereby the narrowness of the ground available to be occupied by a female response to mental pain, as against the space already occupied by succeeding male writers' articulations of masculine melancholy, its causes and its consequences. While Robert Burton, for one, accepts the possibility of female melancholia, especially in 'noble virgins and nice gentlewomen, such as are solitary and idle', nevertheless, as Bridget Gellert Lyons pointed out many years ago, the dramatic representation of melancholy in women was more legitimated in terms of recent widowhood or, as in *The Duchess of Malfi*, of loss of family, while male melancholia could claim a wide range of modes, images and outcomes across the full range of the Renaissance stage.[25] The journey, in the representation of female suffering, from Ophelia to Pope's 'Cave of *Spleen*' with her hand-maids '*Ill-nature*' and '*Affectation*' might have taken more than a century to complete, but the ground covered was, as the crow flies, very little. The two women to whom I turn now, and who attempted in very different ways to write about their troubles of mind, inhabited that ground and made what they could of it, in constructing and reconstructing their depression.

The playwright Sarah Kane, whose tragic suicide took place in February 1999, is quoted in one of her obituaries as having observed: 'Through being very, very low comes an ability to live in the moment because there isn't anything else.'[26] If Boswell both lived and re-lived the moments of his life, depressive and otherwise, Hannah Allen lived in her moments in a rather more restrictive, if equally intense, way. Her pamphlet, *A Narrative of God's Gracious Dealings With That Choice Christian Mrs. Hannah Allen*, which was published in 1683, is an exemplary account of the ways of God in testing and reclaiming a sinner. It is also, more personally, a negotiation of depressive moments, both in the immediacy of their being lived and understood, and in the narrative perspective which subsequently assimilates them, and ultimately therefore denies them, in the context of 'God's Gracious Dealings'. Born in Snelston in Derbyshire as Hannah Archer, she married a merchant, Hannibal Allen, in 1655 and, during the approximately eight years of their marriage, bore one son by him. Hannibal, however, was frequently absent on lengthy trading voyages, and it was his eventual death 'beyond sea' that apparently precipitated her breakdown into depression, or, as she puts it,

I began to fall into deep Melancholy, and no sooner did this black humour begin to darken my Soul, but the Devil set on his former Temptations,... with great strugglings and fightings within me; as I would express it (to my Aunt) I am just as if two were fighting within me, but I trust, the Devil will never be able to overcome me.[27]

Even here, Allen is able to validate her experience through the model of the bereaved widow as well as the tested Christian, thereby trusting in an outcome that inevitably draws the sting from the remorseless presence of the lived-in moment. But as the narrative proceeds, with depression more and more pervasive, the thread of 'God's Gracious Dealings' becomes increasingly stretched as moment after recollected moment insists upon its non-narrative totality. Continuity, for example, is threatened by intervention of the diary form:

The sixth of *April* 64. The truth is I know not well what to say, for as yet I am under sad Melancholy, and sometimes dreadful Temptations, to have hard thoughts of my dearest Lord ... Temptations to impatience and despair, and to give up all for lost; and to close with the Devil and forsake my God, which the Almighty for Christ's sake forbid.[28]

Sentence structure and tense become strained as the narrative attempts to deal with the narrowing in of Allen's linguistic competence, her increasing entrapment within the language of the moment.

After this I writ no more.... I soon after fell into deep Despair, and my language and condition grew sadder than before. Now little to be heard from me, but lamenting my woful state, in very sad and dreadful Expressions; As that I was undone for ever; that I was worse than *Cain* or *Judas*; that now the Devil had overcome me irrecoverably; that this was what he had been aiming at all along; Oh the Devil hath so deceiv'd me as never any one was deceived; he made me believe my condition was good when I was a cursed Hypocrite.[29]

'There isn't anything else', and what is more there never has been anything else. What is now is what had always been intended. The language of now is the only language of truth, and Allen, at the height of her despair, finds her own lived truth in a self-selected model, adopted almost with last-ditch relish, and repeated obsessively, not the widow, not the tested Christian, but the '*Monster of the Creation*':

I would say that *Pashurs* doom belonged to me, that I was *Magor-Missabib*, a Terrour to my self and all my Friends; that I was a Hell upon Earth, and a Devil incarnate;... *I would often say, I was a thousand times worse than the Devil, for the Devil had never committed such Sins as I had; for I had committed worse Sins than the Sin against the Holy-Ghost:... My Sins are so great, that if all the Sins of all the Devils and Damned in Hell, and all the Reprobates on Earth were comprehended in one man; mine are greater; There is no word comes so near the comprehension of the dread-fulness of my Condition; as that, I am the Monster of the Creation:* in this word *I* much delighted.[30]

It is that recollected delight that gives the life to Hannah Allen's moments. Linguistically the force of the pamphlet is there in the series of moments that constitute her depression, that can conceive of no 'later' when, safely restored to 'Choice' Christianity, and safely remarried to 'one Mr. *Charles Hatt*,... my husband being one that truly fears God', she will be able to reconstruct *A Narrative of God's Gracious Dealings* that makes a different sense from there not being anything else. Assimilation back into marriage and God is a register of the disjunction in Allen's narrative. The prolonged absence of her first husband, widowhood, depression, living through that long series of moments between 1663 and 1666 that

culminated in her delight in that self-selected metaphor for her own supposed sinfulness, '*the Monster of the Creation*', these are oblique to the
reintroduction and reaffirmation of a gendered, male perspective on her
experience: the authority of 'blessed Mr. *Bolton*'s Books' that 'so much com-
forted and strengthened' her – this being the popular puritan writer and
preacher, Richard Bolton, who died in 1631; the agreement with her
'Cousin *Walker*' that she would 'believe better of my self, if Mr. *Baxter* told
me my condition was safe' – 'Mr. *Baxter*' is the famous contemporary
Nonconformist divine; the intervention of her friend, the local minister
John Shorthose, who through his advices and his 'some skill in Physick'
found 'means to do me much good both in Soul and Body'.[31] That which
has made for narrative, for continuation and understanding the moments,
has saved Hannah Allen for God and mankind, but has thereby safely
sealed off those lived moments where she chose to express her 'inexpressibly dreadful' self as '*the Monster of the Creation*'.

The ground inhabited by Anne Finch was in most respects diametrically
opposite to Hannah Allen's. Well-born, well and happily married to a
husband, Colonel Heneage Finch, who outlived her, their displacement
from royal circles with the deposition of James II in 1688 was eventually
resolved by a home at Eastwell Park in Kent with Finch's nephew the Earl of
Winchilsea, whom Finch succeeded in 1712. Her depression, however, was
apparently temperamental and life-long, and required periodic visits to the
spa reports such as Tunbridge Wells and Astrop. Suffering neither the losses
of Lady Mary Lane nor the self-recriminations of Hannah Allen, neither a
model of patient endurance nor a monster of creation, Anne Finch's poetry,
written from around 1685 onwards, constitutes her negotiations with
depression, conducted and reconducted over a variety of forms and continuities, a running dialogue of the moments that constitute a lifetime.

Like many other melancholiacs of her time, male and female, the basis of
Finch's gloom is readily expressible. Capable of cheerfulness, playfulness
and variety in her poetry, nevertheless the melancholy vision is perpetually
waiting to re-exert itself whenever she looks about her, its truths apparently
undeniably valid.

> But oh! this God, the Glorious Architect
> Of this fair World

she complains in 'Some Reflections: In a Dialogue Between Teresa and
Ardelia' (her half-sister and intimate friend Dorothy Ogle and herself,
respectively),

> Seems those who trust him most, most to neglect,
> Else me Teresa, else, how could itt be,
> That all his storms attend, and tempests fall on me.

> The Proud he hates, yett me he does expose
> Empty of all things, naked to their scorn.
> His world, on them he liberally bestows,
> Theirs are his Vines, his feilds, his flocks, his corn,
> And all that can sustain, and all that can adorn.[32]

Again, in 'All Is Vanity', which is loosely based on Juvenal's tenth satire, she runs through the forms of life available to those who seek to evade the fundamental truth of human existence: that man is *'ordain'd to Dye!'* and only 'The Architect of Heaven' offers any opportunity for spiritual hope.[33] The pattern is picked up in 'Life's Progress', but here that hope is gone. We begin with expectations –

> How gayly is at first begun
> Our *Life's* uncertain Race!
> Whilst yet that sprightly Morning Sun,
> With which we just set out to run
> Enlightens all the Place.[34]

– only to conclude unfailingly in despair, relieved to be rid of a burdensome existence:

> Till with succeeding Ills opprest
> For Joys we hop'd to find;
> By Age too, rumpl'd and undrest,
> We gladly sinking down to rest,
> Leave following Crouds behind.[35]

If these are some of the traditional complaints of the melancholy man seeking grounds for his melancholy, they nevertheless take on a more overwhelming aspect for Finch, in whose depression poetic negotiation is in perpetual danger of being suppressed by the disabling potency of her vision. The paradox of melancholy in her poetry is that the very vehicle of negotiation, the process that seems to make depression liveable, is always moving towards the point where nothing is worth saying any more, where 'there isn't anything at all'. In 'The Consolation' she seeks for comfort in natural forms – 'See, Phoebus Breaking from the willing skies,/See, how the soaring Lark, does with him rise' – but reveals in 'The Change' that those very forms themselves hold melancholy resonances, both inherently and, here, politically:

> Poor *River*, now thou'rt almost dry,
> What Nymph, or Swain, will near thee lie?...

> And thou, poor *Sun!* that sat'st on high;
> But late, the Splendour of the Sky;
> What Flow'r tho' by thy Influence born,
> Now Clouds prevail, will tow'rds thee turn?[36]

Poetic forms are equally vulnerable. They both express the depressive moment and succumb to it. 'O'er me alas! thou dost too much prevail', she cries in 'The Spleen',

> I feel thy Force, while I against thee rail;
> I feel my Verse decay, and my crampt Numbers fail.
> Thro' thy black Jaundice I all objects see,
>   As Dark, and Terrible as Thee....[37]

The process of negotiation is witnessed in 'Some Reflections: In A Dialogue': arrested in her 'pernitious' complaints against God's favours to 'the Proud' by Teresa, who reminds her of Christ's sacrifice, Ardelia confesses:

> Teresa, from my guilty dream, I wake,
>   The truth has reach'd me, and my fault I find,
> Forgive me God, forgive the short mistake,...
>
> I saw the Mighty, and began to slide,
>   My feet were gone, but I return again.... [38]

Under pressure, poetry could not hold: external reassurance enters the negotiation, preventing the slide, finding her feet. But in 'Ardelia to Melancholy' there is no external reassurance, only Finch addressing her depression and submitting:

> At last, my old inveterate foe,
> No opposition shalt thou know.
> Since I by struggling, can obtain
> Nothing, but encrease of pain,
> I will att last, no more do soe,...

She has fought; music, mirth, friendship have proved vain, and even, finally, poetry:

> These failing, I invok'd a Muse,
> And Poetry wou'd often use,
> To guard me from the Tyrant pow'r;
> And to oppose thee ev'ry hour

New troops of fancy's, did I chuse.
Alas! in vain, for all agree
To yeild me Captive up to thee,
And heav'n, alone, can sett me free.[39]

Here is the last possible statement: not a negotiation any more, but the complete surrender that ends the poem.

Yet there are other poems. All closures are provisional because depression remits and recurs. Wherever and whatever, it is always there, waiting within the moments. As she begins in exasperation 'The Spleen':

What art thou, *SPLEEN*, which ev'ry thing dost ape?
Thou *Proteus* to abus'd Mankind,
Who never yet thy real Cause cou'd find,
Or fix thee to remain in one continued Shape.[40]

Problematically, spleen is everything and nothing, capable of being addressed, negotiated, confronted in an endless series of forms but never concluded with, never yielding a final truth, never ultimately expressible. Narrative is impossible. God's dealings are never conclusively gracious, no Christian is ever unproblematically choice. There are only poetry and depression, in uneasy relation to each other, only a series of lived-in moments.

By 1793, Boswell was resident in London. Several hundred miles away, in Scotland, Andrew Erskine, Boswell's life-long friend and fellow hypochondriac, finally gave up his struggle against depression. The news of Erskine's suicide was entered into Boswell's journal: he had received, he said, 'an intimation from Sir William Forbes that my old friend _____ had killed himself'.[41] Boswell and Erskine, when young, had published together, including the playful *Letters Between the Honourable Andrew Erskine and James Boswell, Esq*. Later letters, not written for publication, had contributed to the safe confession of hypochondriac suffering, evidence of a relationship which was founded upon the word. But here, in the blank that Boswell could not fill, where Andrew Erskine's name should be, we read a fitting testimony to the man with whom depressive intimacies had been shared, and a fitting epitaph on the language of confession. Identity has been reduced to anonymity, feeling to emptiness. Reality is elsewhere, beyond the confessional word, while the language that once apparently gave truth and life, that redeemed from oblivion, is replaced by a confessional space.

James Boswell was above all a creature of language, one whose whole being had to exist in language before it could properly be said to exist. For the written word to fail him at last is evidence that, by the end of his life, his depression had indeed become 'inexpressibly dreadful'. The cases of Hannah Allen and Anne Finch are dissimilar, the forms of expression differently constituted, the depressions differently handled and constructed. But neither was ready to assume the role that apparently suited Lady Mary Lane and her admiring dedicator, Timothy Rogers, who staked out the territory of the male melancholiac. What Allen and Finch have in common, through their differences, is the genuineness of an individual female voice speaking for herself, irrespective of who owns the land, and the grim isolation of that voice, surviving within her depression.

Notes

1   Timothy Rogers, *A Discourse Concerning Trouble of Mind and the Disease of Melancholly* (1691), in *Patterns of Madness in the Eighteenth Century: A Reader*, ed. Allan Ingram (Liverpool, 1998), p. 37.
2   Rogers, p. 37.
3   Rogers, pp. 37–8.
4   James Boswell, *Boswell's Column (The Hypochondriack)*, ed. Margery Bailey (London, 1951), p. 336.
5   James Boswell, *Boswell: The Ominous Years, 1774–1776*, ed. Charles Ryskamp and F. A. Pottle (London, 1963), p. 265.
6   James Boswell, *Boswell in Holland, 1763–1764*, ed. F. A. Pottle (London, 1952), p. 206.
7   Philip Martin, *A Life of James Boswell* (London, 1999), p. 20.
8   James Boswell, *Private Papers of James Boswell from Malahide Castle*, ed. Geoffrey Scott and F. A. Pottle, 18 volumes (New York, 1928–34) vol. 16, p. 202.
9   Boswell, *Private Papers*, vol. 16, p. 203 and vol. 15, p. 105.
10 Boswell, *Ominous Years*, p. 214.
11 For this and the entries of 1 and 2 December, see James Boswell, *Boswell in Extremes, 1776–1778*, ed. Charles McC. Weis and F. A. Pottle (London, 1971), pp. 61–3.
12 Boswell, *Boswell in Extremes*, pp. 64–5.
13 James Boswell, *Boswell's London Journal, 1762–1763*, ed. F. A. Pottle (London, 1951), p. 74.
14 Boswell, *Boswell's London Journal*, p. 211.
15 Boswell, *Boswell in Extremes*, p. 102.
16 Boswell, *Ominous Years*, p. 306.
17 Boswell, *London Journal*, p. 229.
18 Boswell, *Boswell's Column*, p. 325.
19 Boswell, *London Journal*, p. 67.
20 Boswell, *Ominous Years*, p. 240.
21 Boswell, *Holland*, p. 207.
22 Boswell, *Private Papers*, vol. 18, p. 70–1.
23 Boswell, *Private Papers*, vol. 18, p. 66.
24 Boswell, *Private Papers*, vol. 17, p. 47.
25 Robert Burton, *The Anatomy of Melancholy* (1621), ed. H. Jackson (London, 1964) vol. 1, p. 417; Bridget Gellert Lyons, *Voices of Melancholy: Studies in Literary Treatments of Melancholy in Renaissance England* (London, 1971), p. 55.
26 Lyn Gardner, 'Sarah Kane: Obituary', *The Guardian*, Tuesday, 23 February, 1999, p. 16.
27 Hannah Allen, *A Narrative of God's Gracious Dealings With that Choice Christian Mrs. Hannah Allen* (1683), ed. Allan Ingram, *Voices of Madness: Four Pamphlets*, 1683–1796 (Stroud, 1997), p. 6.

28 Allen, p. 8.
29 Allen, p. 9.
30 Allen, p. 13.
31 Allen, pp. 6, 16, 19.
32 Ingram, *Patterns*, pp. 57–8.
33 Anne Finch, *The Poems of Anne Finch Countess of Winchilsea*, ed. Myra Reynolds (Chicago, 1903), pp. 247–48.
34 Finch, p. 136.
35 Finch, p. 138.
36 Finch, pp.18, 84.
37 Ingram, *Patterns*, pp. 60–1.
38 Finch, p. 225.
39 Ingram, *Patterns*, p. 55.
40 Ingram, *Patterns*, p. 59.
41 Boswell, *Private Papers*, vol. 18, p. 221.

6
Wonders in the Deep: Cowper, Melancholy and Religion[1]

Stephen Sykes

Virtually by definition a mental illness for a person of religious faith involves a crisis of faith. The reason is not difficult to understand. In the case of Christianity, for example, believers are taught that God loves the world and humankind, that there is point and purpose to their existence, and that it is possible for them to know and to do God's will. And quite apart from hearing and believing the teaching (in part) most believers will have had some kind of confirmatory experiences, or have attempted to interpret life experiences in a confirmatory way. 'O taste and see how gracious the Lord is' is a verse from the Hebrew Psalter (34.8) regularly applied to the way in which Christians approach prayer and worship.

Under conditions of mental illness some or all of these Christian teachings and experiences seem false. God may appear to be malicious and punitive, the world process inexplicable, and one's own part in it absurd or destructive. Plenty of Christians or people with Christian backgrounds have come to draw some or all of these conclusions under conditions of severe mental illness, and something closely analogous occurs in other belief-systems. Ignoring this crisis is to fail to treat a whole person; imposing a form of reductive rationalism upon sufferers is a species of bullying akin to abuse. A humane psychiatry has to find a way of taking seriously the religious faith of people presenting with mental illnesses. It has a duty to help them find a way of regrouping and of reassembling those forms of life-meaning which most assist the processes and techniques of coping. And the obvious first port of call ought to be the resources of the specific religion professed by the sufferer.

This paper concerns the religion, the illness and the marvellous literary activity of William Cowper (1731–1800), an eighteenth-century Christian, member of the Church of England, and evangelical. It is a story of creativity as a refuge from or antidote to madness, rather than one of creative madness. Its context concerns the history, literature and psychiatric practices of the eighteenth century, but with an extra dimension, namely religion – and not merely religion in its expansive modern guise as 'spirituality', but a highly specific form of evangelical Calvinism. Did Cowper suffer from 'religious mania' of an extreme kind, the short-hand term adopted by Peter Ackroyd in his recent biography of William Blake?[2] My argument is that this verdict is unsatisfactory and even misleading in part. What Cowper's life displays most powerfully is the experience of a Christian of Calvinist convictions regrouping his life-meaning out of the crises of his episodes of illness. Cowper most typically copes on the basis of the resources of Christian faith, together with the kindness and good intentions (and despite the occasional stupidities) of his friends – much as any contemporary is obliged to do. What distinguishes Cowper is his genius with words, his directness, his insight into his condition, his wit and the attractive gentleness of his character.

We shall see that writing was for him a self-administered therapy, which kept melancholy at bay, or within bounds. But it was not an infallible remedy, and Cowper's last six years of life were years of virtually unrelieved depression. Even so he was occasionally well enough to write, and twelve months before his death he composed 'The Castaway', ostensibly about a sailor who was washed overboard and left to drown, but finishing with a stunning stanza of self-reference:

> No voice divine the storm allay'd,
>   No light propitious shone,
> When, snatch'd from all effectual aid,
>   We perish'd, each, alone;
> But I, beneath a rougher sea,
> And whelm'd in deeper gulphs than he.[3]

Are these lines really to be read as 'Cowper's final considered and terrible judgement on his own life', as Lord David Cecil held in his brilliant but flawed biography?[4] I shall propose a different reading, based on a different view of Cowper's relationship with the resources of his faith. There is, I shall suggest, a more dialectical way of interpreting these lines, as a kind of counter-point to biblical passages well-known to Cowper, especially passages from the Book of Psalms, which is rich in references to 'wonders in the deep' (Ps107:24).[5] This paper will seek to show how the springs of Cowper's creativity were enriched by the very religious traditions which at the same time were deeply problematic to him.

Cowper is somewhat in danger of being defined by the episodes of acute illness which he occasionally endured. The recent Everyman edition of his works (1999) starts with the five stanzas entitled 'Lines Written During a Period of Insanity', with 'The Cast-Away' placed second.[6] (This, together with the lowering cover-illustration, courtesy of Superstock, suggests that the association of creativity with madness has marketing potential.) But we should insist that Cowper was well for long periods of time. In the 1770s and 1780s he had more than a decade of extraordinary productivity.[7] Furthermore, he was perfectly capable of seeing the funny side of life in circumstances far from comfortable, as he does in the delightful poem about being stuck in mud whilst out for a walk with a friend, Mrs Mary Unwin – a poem thought by Hayley to be too frivolous for publication.[8]

King and Ryskamp state that Cowper suffered from no less than five 'periods of depression'.[9] The first is dated November 1753, when Cowper was a 22-year-old in love with his cousin Theadora, and in residence in the Middle Temple. The source of the information is Cowper himself, in his autobiographical sketch of his life and his brother's life and death up to 1772. Here he speaks of being struck by an acute 'dejection of spirits' and of being on the rack, 'lying down in horror and rising in despair'.[10] In the end relief came, he records, from the beauty of a day spent by the sea near the New Forest. A poem in the following year written to Robert Lloyd, one of his group of able and boisterous ex-Westminster friends in the Nonsense Club (the 'London Geniuses', as Boswell called them), already makes clear the benefits he derives from the act of writing poetry. He composes, he explains,

> ...to divert a fierce banditti,
> (Sworn foes to every thing that's witty!),
> That, with a black, infernal train,
> Make cruel inroads in my brain,
> And daily threaten to drive thence
> My little garrison of sense:
> The fierce banditti, which I mean,
> Are gloomy thoughts led on by spleen.[11]

About this time his uncle, Ashley Cowper, prohibited the marriage of William and Theadora, and there is ample but confusing evidence of how difficult William found this ban.

The first, indubitable and absolutely major crisis of his life was vividly described by Cowper in the autobiography, *Adelphi*, already mentioned. The story of his repeated attempts at committing suicide after having been offered in 1763 (at age 32) a minor administrative post in the House of Lords, of his being conveyed to a *Collegium Insanorum* in St Albans, of his treatment, religious conversion and recovery, is so precise and detailed[12] as to be accessible to contemporary diagnosis. Dr Pauline Watson has provided a professional psychiatric view of his condition in the following terms:

> From [the *Adelphi* account], a modern psychiatrist would be very likely to diagnose him as suffering from a severe depressive episode with psychotic symptoms.[13]

Watson writes further:

> He is agitated and restless, preoccupied by thoughts of suicide but ambivalent about carrying it out. The degree of distress and depression he was feeling is shown in the preceding section, when he is considering whether suicide can be a morally acceptable option. He feels that even if this were not the case but he proceeded to commit suicide, then everlasting suffering in Hell could not be worse that his present predicament.
>
> At this stage he has delusions of persecution, believing that articles in the newspaper are satires on him.... He is concerned that his thoughts can be known by others, demonstrating his loss of a sense of clear boundary between himself and the rest of the world. He has a delusional belief that Satan is urging him to suicide. All his thinking is preoccupied with his fear of going to the House of Lords, the need to escape and his possible suicide. He wakes at 3am and has distressing dreams, both typical symptoms of depression. He describes being 'decent' on the outside but full of rottenness within. He feels so desperate that he overcomes his ambivalence and attempts suicide several times.
>
> After the attempted hanging, there is a sudden crystallising out of his feeling of rottenness into further explanatory delusional beliefs of sin and wickedness. This for the time being gives him some relief from his suicidal impulses but only because of his strong sense of sin and guilt about his attempts and the subsequent conviction that he will be damned to everlasting punishment if he dies.
>
> He describes this conviction of sin as 'unbelievably strong' – this has the fixed, unshakable quality of a delusion and he cannot listen to attempts to modify his view or be comforted. His agitation continues, 'he paces to and fro' and searches religious literature for relief. However, he finds only confirmation of his sin. Further ideas of reference: 'I found something in every author to condemn me.' There are 'sleepless nights and uninterrupted misery'.
>
> He has a belief in a harsh, punishing God but one whom he also idealises. He believes that God has given him this insight into his sin as a means of attempting to do 'quickening work' with him. Any loving and forgiving aspects of God have been eliminated by this delusional distortion.
>
> He describes ongoing paranoid delusions that people laugh at him and hold him in contempt. There is evidence of thought broadcasting: 'my conscience was loud enough for everybody to hear it', and he avoids people for these reasons. Any attempt to distract himself is followed by

renewed self-chastisement. He looks back over his life and concentrates on misdemeanours, which he magnifies as further evidence of his great sin. This 'retrospective distortion' is characteristic of depression. He tries to gain consolation from prayer, but when he is unable to remember the words, he misinterprets this in a delusional way. When he fails to profess his faith in the Holy Ghost, this he 'considered as a supernatural interposition to inform me that I had sinned against the Holy Ghost...I delivered myself to despair'.

All this, the unrelenting distress, agitation, sleep disturbance, bad dreams, depressed mood, preoccupation with anxiety and self-blame, delusions (mainly congruent with his depressed mood) of sin, guilt and persecution and intense suicidal wishes are symptoms of a severe psychotic depressive illness.

The pattern of his illness with five episodes throughout his adult life, provoked by a variety of stresses or losses, is typical of a recurrent depression. The last episode was very prolonged and he did not make a proper recovery before his death – this is a common pattern with depression, which is more difficult to treat in older people.[14]

Adelphi was based on a memoir Cowper had written in 1767, two years after leaving the 'Collegium Insanorum'. It is remarkable enough that Cowper recalls his confinement there without animus. He needed to be restrained; he was, he said, carefully watched; and there was at least one attendant ('one of the profanest wretches in the world') who attracted his antipathy. But for Nathaniel Cotton, the physician, he had nothing but admiration. Particularly striking was his willingness to talk with Cowper, to tell him funny stories, and after his recovery to join him daily in spiritual conversation ('the Gospel was always the delightful theme').[15] Cowper realised how fortunate he was in both respects, and wrote (in 1765) in the following terms to his cousin:

I was not only treated by him with the greatest tenderness, while I was ill, and attended with the utmost diligence, but when my reason was restored to me, and I had so much need of a religious friend to converse with, to whom I could open my mind upon the subject without reserve, I could hardly have found a fitter person for the purpose. My eagerness and anxiety to settle my opinions upon that long neglected point, made it necessary that while my mind was yet weak, and my spirits uncertain, I should have some assistance. The Doctor was as ready to administer relief to me in this article likewise, and as well qualified to do it as in that which was more immediately his province. How many physicians would have thought this an irregular appetite, and a symptom of remaining madness! But if it were so, my friend was as mad as myself, and it is well for me that he was so.[16]

The reputation of eighteenth century psychiatry, including that of private asylums, was quite other. Sir Richard Steele had written some sixty years earlier:

> I took three Lads who are under my Guardianship a rambling in a Hackney-coach, to show 'em the Town, as the Lions, the Tombs, Bedlam, and the other Places which are entertainment to raw minds, because they strike forcibly on the fancy.[17]

William Hogarth, who became a Governor of Bedlam, included a 'Scene in a Madhouse' as the last episode of his *Rake's Progress* (1733). This pitiful scene containing:

> Shapes of Horror, that wou'd even
> Cast Doubt of Mercy upon Heaven.[18]

has nonetheless the aspect of a Deposition from the Cross, as Jenny Uglow observes in her magnificent study of William Hogarth. The scene has a double character; it places Christian theology in doubt, while at the same time reminding one that the suffering of Christ lies at its heart.[19]

On his recovery Cowper headed for Huntingdon, the nearest lodging he could find to Cambridge, where his brother, a fellow of Corpus Christi (then called Bene't College), lived. Here he had the good fortune to form a friendship with the Unwin family. On Morley Unwin's death, Cowper moved together with Mary, his widow, to Olney, near Northampton, in order to be close to the Evangelical convert and parish curate, John Newton. Encouraged by Newton, William Cowper now contributed to a collection of hymns evidently sung at more or less informal church gatherings, and eventually published by Newton as *Olney Hymns* (February 1779).[20] This group of hymns, with *Adelphi* and the letters of that period, represent the high point of Cowper's conviction that his life was governed by God's providential care. In the light of what was to come it is particularly poignant that among these hymns is a direct reflection upon the mystery of divine providence entitled *Light Shining Out of Darkness*:

> God moves in a mysterious way,
> His wonders to perform,
> He plants his footsteps in the Sea,
> And rides upon the Storm.
>
> Deep in unfathomable Mines,
> Of never failing Skill,
> He treasures up his bright designs,
> And works his Sovereign Will.

Ye fearfull Saints fresh courage take,
The clouds ye so much dread,
Are big with Mercy, and shall break
In blessings on your head.

Judge not the Lord by feeble sense,
But trust him for his Grace,
Behind a frowning Providence
He hides a Smiling face.

His purposes will ripen fast,
Unfolding every hour,
The Bud may have a bitter taste,
But *wait*, to *Smell the flower*.

Blind unbelief is sure to err,
And scan his work in vain,
God is his own Interpreter,
And he will make it plain.[21]

But by the time that hymn was published, Cowper had already suffered in January and February 1773, at the age of 42, a second major crisis. Fourteen years later, in a letter to his cousin, Lady Hesketh (who was Theadora's sister), he describes his sudden return to a still deeper condition of melancholy than he had endured in St Albans:

I was suddenly reduced from my wonted rate of understanding to an almost childish imbecility. I did not indeed lose my senses, but I lost the power to exercise them. I could return a rational answer even to a difficult question, but a question was necessary, or I never spoke at all. This state of mind was accompanied, as I suppose it to be in most instances of the kind, with misapprehension of things and persons that made me a very untractable patient. I believed that every body hated me, and that Mrs. Unwin hated me most of all; was convinced that all my food was poisoned, together with ten thousand megrims of the same stamp. I would not be more circumstantial than is necessary. Dr. Cotton was consulted. He replied that he could do no more for me than might be done at Olney, but recommended particular vigilance, lest I should attempt my life: – a caution for which there was the greatest occasion. At the same time that I was convinced of Mrs. Unwin's aversion to me, could endure no other companion. The whole management of me consequently devolved upon her, and a terrible task she had; she performed it, however, with a cheerfulness hardly ever equalled on such an occasion; and I have often heard her say, that if ever she praised God in her life it was when she found that she was to have all the labour.[22]

The account makes clear that Cowper was aware that his mental condition involved delusions or 'misapprehensions'. He also spoke of them as 'nervous fevers' which 'creep silently into the Citadel and put the Garrison to the Sword'.[23] But later, when writing to Newton, his description of what had happened takes on another character:

> I had a dream 12 years ago, before the recollection of which, all consolation vanishes, and, as it seems to me, must always vanish. But I will neither trouble you with my dream nor with any comments upon it, for if it were possible, I should do well to forget that, the remembrance of which is incompatible with my comfort.[24]

That Cowper eventually told Newton the content of this dream, a voice portentously announcing (in Latin) *'Actum est de te, periisti'* ('it's all over with you; you have perished'), is evident from Newton's repetition of the words in his funeral oration on Cowper.[25] We need to examine Newton's peculiar relationship with Cowper shortly, but it is clear that Newton believed that dreams could reveal important truths. In the latter part of Cowper's life, a schoolmaster from Olney, Samuel Teedon, whom Cowper at first regarded as a more than slightly absurd pedant, came to exercise a significant influence over Cowper, specifically in relation to his dreams and nightmares.[26]

The fourth period of depression identified by King and Ryskamp occurred between January and June 1787, when Cowper was 56. It began three months after the sudden death of William Unwin, Mary's son, and one of Cowper's closest friends. Cowper had become famous through the success attending the publication of *The Task* (1785),[27] and Olney became a site of literary pilgrimage. Of the impact on him of his dreams he wrote revealingly to his cousin:

> I have not believed that I shall perish because in dreams I have been told it, but because I have had hardly any but terrible dreams for 13 years, I therefore have spent the greatest part of that time most unhappily. They have either tinged my mind with melancholy or filled it with terrour, and the effect has been unavoidable. If we swallow arsenic we must be poison'd, and he who dreams as I have done, must be troubled. So much for dreams.[28]

It was, he told his friends, to keep melancholy at bay that he wrote poetry.[29] To William Unwin, he claimed that no one in England had written more verse in 1781 than he. Six years later he was reaping the whirlwind. Actors performed John Gilpin up and down the country; Fox and other politicians quoted Cowper in parliamentary speeches; his poems were read at Court; there were resolutions to erect statues in his honour; and a constant stream of requests for comment or patronage arrived at his door. It seems entirely possible that this period of ill health, about which he did not write much, was more akin to exhaustion than to acute depression.

Not so, however, can we interpret Cowper's final afflictions, which grew in intensity from January 1794. In a letter he makes clear that he knows that January is his worst month, and that his spirits generally lighten during the day. He continued to be occasionally capable of work, amazingly beginning a revision of his translation of Homer in November 1797. But most of his letters, particularly to friends who did their best to reassure him, are filled with despair. For Mary Unwin, who had suffered strokes in 1791 and '92, he wrote lines which demonstrated both his affection for her and awareness that his condition influences her own:

> But ah by constant heed I know
> How oft the sadness that I show
> Transforms thy smiles to looks of woe
> My Mary!

> And should my future lot be cast
> With much resemblance of the past,
> Thy worn-out heart will break at last
> My Mary![30]

Mary Unwin died in December 1796. Cowper's friends tried to alleviate his melancholy by means of a change of residence, removal to the Lincolnshire asylum of Dr Francis Willis, King George III's medical adviser, reassuring correspondence from eminent people, and even the absurd device of booming comforting words at night through a tin tube inserted into a partition in Cowper's bedroom. It is true that he believed that he had committed an unforgivable sin; he asserted that the severity of God's judgement on him was wholly disproportionate to his mercy; that if God was really merciful, he would not have made him at all; he spoke of himself as a 'Calvinist from experience', meaning that his mental infirmity had denied him any freedom to choose.[31] This is the immediate psychological background to the poem, 'The Castaway', with its sense of being abandoned by God. Cowper died in 1800, and was buried in East Dereham Church in Norfolk.

The question that immediately occurred to those who reflected on Cowper's sufferings was whether his Evangelical Calvinist beliefs, and those of his friends, contributed to his state of mind. John Newton had the reputation for 'preaching people mad', and critics were quick to point the finger at the spiritually intense relationship he enjoyed with the hypersensitive poet in Olney. In the eighteenth century, the evangelicals both were a force to be reckoned with and provoked huge antipathy. In 1762 William Hogarth published his print *Credulity, Superstition and Fanaticism*. An hysterical non-conformist preacher dangles a witch and a devil from either hand, as his wig flies off to reveal a papist tonsure beneath. The Pauline text, 'I speak as a fool', is complemented by harlequin undergarments and a scale of vociferation at his side measures the volume from natural tone to bull roar, with the words, 'Blood, blood, blood' at the top. Below, perched on a volume of Wesley's Sermons and Glanvil on Witches, is a thermometer of madness, with raving at one end and suicide at the other. The centre of the picture is occupied by a man at a reading desk containing a quotation from Whitefield's hymns, while Whitefield's *Journal* is in the bucket of a shady character spitting nails onto the robe of the notorious Mary Tofts and her rabbits.[32] And over the congregation a candle stand swings menacingly, mapped with the regions of hell and its gaping mouth proclaiming 'Eternal Damnation Gulf'.[33]

Satires of this kind did not distinguish between the rather different theologies of Wesley and Whitefield, and the term 'Methodist' was widely used for all forms of evangelical enthusiasm. Indeed Cowper, who was an Anglican, applied the term to himself. On the other hand both he and Newton had developed their own theological stance, and he knew precisely what he was doing when in 1781, in the poem 'Hope', he explicitly praised and defended the Calvinist, George Whitefield. The same poem also makes clear that Cowper understood the 'terms' on which salvation has been offered to humankind.

> Compliance with his will your lot insures,
> Accept it only, and the boon is yours;
> And sure it is as kind to smile and give,
> As with a frown to say, do this and live.
> Love is not pedlars trump'ry, bought and sold,
> He will give freely, or he will withhold,
> His soul abhors a mercenary thought,
> And him as deeply who abhors it not;
> He stipulates indeed, but merely this,
> That man will freely take an unbought bliss,
> Will trust him for a faithful gen'rous part,
> Nor set a price upon a willing heart.[34]

The poem continues with a gentle poking of fun at various characters who object to the idea that salvation is by grace alone apart from the help of meritorious good works. Cowper had read and enjoyed Fielding's novel, *Joseph Andrews* (1742),[35] and it is Parson Adams' view of Whitefield he has in his sights.

Mention of the term 'Calvinism' of course is enough to evoke the memory of Robert Burns's savage satire in Holy Willie's Prayer:

> O thou that in the heavens does dwell!
> Wha, as it pleases best thysel
> Sends one to heaven, and ten to h-ll,
>   A' for thy glory!
> And no for any gude or ill
>   They've done before thee.[36]

This doctrine of predestination to both salvation and damnation, which nauseatingly permits Willy[37] both to admit fornication and pray for vengeance on his enemies ('And a' the glory shall be thine! AMEN! AMEN!'), is sometimes known as High Calvinism. It was explicitly repudiated by John Newton. A careful examination of his convictions, based on sermons of the 1780s and 1790s, shows clearly that he refused to follow the strict logic of high Calvinism, and preached on the assumption that there was a role for human agency.[38] He both was, and understood himself to be, a moderate, always looking for common ground between evangelicals of different persuasions, and suspicious of abstract principles.

At the same time it is clear that those who had responded to the gospel of grace needed the assurance of inner conviction that they belonged to God's chosen people. The quest for experiential verification, which Max Weber called the *certitudo salutis*, was directly expressed by Cowper in his Olney Hymn, 'The Contrite Heart':

> The Lord will happiness divine
>   On contrite hearts bestow:
> Then tell me, gracious God, is mine
>   A contrite heart or no.[39]

As the hymn continues, based on a passage from Isaiah 57:15 ('I dwell...also with him that is of a contrite and humble spirit'), the author complains that he is 'insensible as steel' and wracked with pain at his lack of feeling. He closes:

> O make this heart rejoice, or ache;
>   Decide this doubt for me;
> And if it be not broken, break,
>   And heal it, if it be.[40]

Dick Watson in his magisterial study, *The English Hymn*, aptly describes this hymn as a 'rare example of a penitential hymn that does not at some point become pleased with itself at being penitent'.[41] This uncertainty about his own experience of salvation is not to be interpreted as a doctrine of salvation by feelings. Newton himself saw inner peace as something variable; he wrote in his diary for 1757 that though assurance might in some respects be of the essence of faith, that did not exclude the experience of doubt or fear. In short, recent research into Newton's type of evangelicalism by no means supports the proposal that Cowper was a victim of grim predestinarian zealotry, as David Cecil suggested.[42] The form in which Cowper embraced Calvinism was moderate and psychologically balanced. The crisis of faith precipitated by his mental illness was both predictable and normal, and it took the form of the eminently sensible question, why on earth was there no rescue or relief from suffering for this devoted believer?

There is, of course, plenty of evidence that Cowper himself both asked and attempted to answer that question for himself, and one way of interpreting that evidence is to speak, with Vincent Newey, of Cowper's 'outright acceptance in "The Castaway" of the fact that he has perished inwardly and spiritually' and of a 'concomitant acceptance of a life and a world *without God*'.[43] But my proposal is that we qualify that judgement by noting the audiences for whom Cowper wrote his most far-reaching negations. It is, in my view, of some importance that those in relation to whom he was most insistent on the hopelessness of his predicament were those who made the most strenuous efforts to reassure him.

John Newton is the outstanding example of a partner in dialogue, and in this case we have to do with someone who had also seen Newton at his suicidal worst. Newton left Olney in 1780 to become rector of St Mary, Woolnoth in London. Letters to Newton and separately to his wife begin from 6 February 1780. On 3 May, Cowper depicts himself as a 'man that expects hereafter to be imprisoned in a dungeon where nothing but misery and deformity are to be found'.[44] On 10 May, doubtless in response to some encouraging message, he writes:

> That a Calvinist in principle, should know himself to have been Elected, and yet believe that he is lost, is indeed a Riddle, and so obscure that it Sounds like a Solecism in terms, and may well bring the asserter of it under the Suspicion of Insanity.[45]

After a summer of correspondence Cowper returns on 24 September to the same theme, raised for him by contact with the minister of an independent chapel in Newport Pagnall, the Reverend William Bull. This man doubtless also had attempted to offer spiritual encouragement. The letter is all the more important for the clear distinctions drawn between the various partners with whom Cowper is in contact.

> The short remainder of my Life, the beginning of which was spent in Sin, and the latter part of which has been poisoned with Despair, must

be trifled away in Amusements which I despise too much to be entertained with; or sacrificed at the foot of a regret which can know neither End or abatement. I am conversible upon any Topic but the only one which He would wish to converse upon, and being condemned to a state which I in vain endeavor to describe, because it is incredible, I am out of the reach of consolation, and am indeed a fit Companion for Nobody. If Mrs. Unwin attempts to encourage me, and tells me there is Hope, I can bear it with some degree of Patience, but I can do no more. From her however I can endure it, either because I have been long accustom'd to such language from her Lips, or because it is impossible for any thing that she speaks to give me pain. But I should be otherwise affected by the same things spoken by Mr. Bull; and all that he would gain by conversing with me would be summed up in a single word, astonishment. He would wonder that a Man whose views on the Scripture are just like his own, who is a Calvinist from experience, and knows his election, should be furnished with a Shield of despair impenetrable to every argument by which he might attempt to comfort him. But so it is, and in the end it will be accounted for.[46]

It is exactly the same sentiment when, in a letter to Mrs Newton a few days later (5 October 1780), he pours out a thought about it being better to be swallowed up in the ocean than to be scribbling away quietly as he does – and then apologises by saying that he is irresistibly drawn to such expressions when writing to her or her husband.[47] It is plain, then, that there is a dialectic at work between affirmation and negation, and that Cowper was conscious of using specific people in this way.

It is at this point that I wish to propose that one must take into account when dealing with a writer like Cowper steeped in the study of the Bible, that this resource itself is patterned by affirmation and negation. The most obvious and extensive example is the Book of Job, with its stark juxtaposition of incompatible perspectives from the sufferer and his comforters. But it is the Psalms, with their repeated evocation of storms, deeps, floods, waters and waves, which provide the richest resource for the discourse of drowning, or of being overwhelmed, on the one hand, and of quietening or rescue on the other.[48] Most of these contain both the crisis and its reversal. In Psalm 42 the one who complains, 'all thy waves and storms are gone over me' (v. 9), utters the reassurance at the end, 'O put thy trust in God: for I will yet thank him, which is the help of my countenance and my God' (v. 15). But an example of unrelieved complaint is Psalm 88, 'Thou has laid me in the lowest pit: in a place of darkness, and on the deep. Thine indignation lieth hard upon me: and thou hast vexed me with all thy storms' (vv. 5–6).

In relation specifically to 'The Castaway' Vincent Newey rightly reminds us that much of the 'herio-romantic' language of the poem is to be found in Pope's rendering of Homer's Odyssey.[49] But another resource, surely, is the Book of Psalms, which, quite specifically unlike the respite afforded to Ulysses, is capable of confronting the divine with the absence of rescue.

> Lord, why abhorrest thou my soul:
> and hidest thou thy face from me?
> I am in misery, and like unto him that is at the point to die:
> even from my youth up thy terrors have I suffered with a troubled mind.
> Thy wrathful displeasure goeth over me:
> and the fear of thee hath undone me (Ps 88.14–16).

Cowper's capacity is to write well in great distress. 'The Castaway' is a kind of triumph and we should note that, for good measure, Cowper composed a Latin version of it as well. Newey rightly insists:

> Far from shunning the horror of his situation as 'destin'd wretch' and the inimical darkness of a world from which God (a *deus absconditus*) and all hope are absent, Cowper takes hold of them, from first to last, with deliberateness, zest, and sensitivity that raise him well above mere pessimism, self-pity, or blank despair.[50]

But in order to achieve this 'creative and psychological strength', Newey has Cowper progressively take leave of the God in whom he once believed. In my view, the resources of the Christian faith Cowper embraced included expressions of dereliction, in which the dialect was unexpressed but implicit.[51] Even the despairing-sounding verdict which expresses the central religious problem of his life, why 'no voice divine the storm allayed',[52] is a reference to Jesus' saying to the tempest the words, 'Peace, be still' (Mark 4:38). The best sense that Cowper made of this absence was to propose that God had chosen him to bear this appalling suffering. The biblical resources on which he drew enabled him to affirm this, without mitigation, as a negative pole that was a counterpoint to the affirmation of his friends.

In saying this I am aware that it might not be so. It is proper to ask how Cowper could have ever expressed the sense of God's absence or non-existence, that he was truly alone in a God-less universe, without some cheerful soul later offering the comfortable gloss that his was but one side of a dialectic. We should note that Cowper is not the first or the last example of a religious person confronted and dismayed by great pain or suffering. Wilfred Owen in the First World War is another case of a writer presenting a biblically-phrased protest against facile religiosity.[53] And I have visited this place myself.

So I do not profess to know with any certainty the state of Cowper's mind in his final years. But at least there is no necessity either to regard his as a wholly exceptional case of 'religious mania' (Ackroyd), or to assert that he finally concluded that his earlier beliefs were mistaken (Newey), let alone to view his complex struggle to make spiritual sense of his world as in some way defined by the most negative expression of it.

The interpreter of Cowper is personally confronted with making sense of that suffering, as were Cowper's friends and contemporaries. I embrace a faith which knows of a time and place where someone said, 'My God, my God, why hast thou forsaken me' (Matt 27.46; Mark 15.34). That too was a quotation from the Book of Psalms; and that Psalm also contains the words, 'he hath not hid his face from him, but when he called unto him, he heard him' (Ps 22:1 and 24).

Notes

1   I am grateful for the assistance of Ms Laura L. Brenneman in the preparation of this paper.
2   See Peter Ackroyd, *Blake* (London, 1995), p. 222.
3   From John D. Baird and Charles Ryskamp, eds., *The Poems of William Cowper*, vol. 3 (Oxford, 1995), p. 216.
4   Lord David Cecil, *The Stricken Deer* (London, 1933), p. 298.
5   I do not pretend that Cowper's sufferings were not real and persistent, or that his Calvinist convictions had no resonance with his sense of abandonment. But there are at the very least puzzles about Cowper's relationship with his faith and the friends who tried to offer him consolation.
6   Michael Bruce, ed., *William Cowper*, Everyman's Poetry (London, 1999).
7   Including 'The Diverting History of John Gilpin', which is found in *Poems*, vol. 2 (Oxford, 1995), pp. 295–303. It was said, of course, that the original story was told him in order to prevent him from sinking 'into increasing dejection' (from William Hayley, *Memoirs of the Life and Writing of William Hayley Esq.* Vol. 2 (1823), pp. 128–9; cited in *Poems*, vol. 2, p. 436).
8   'The Distressed Travellers, or Labour in Vain', from *Poems*, vol. 2, p. 13.
9   From James King and Charles Ryskamp, eds., *The Letters and Prose Writings of William Cowper*, vol. 1 (Oxford, 1979), pp. xix–xxii.
10   From Cowper's *Adelphi*, reproduced in *Letters*, vol. 1, p. 8. He describes finding delight in reading George Herbert's verse, until advised by a relative that it was likely to be bad for him (p. 9).
11   *Poems*, vol 1, p. 55.
12   As described in *Letters*, vol. 1, pp. 39–40; see also Cowper's account of this in a letter to his cousin, Lady Hesketh (*Letters*, vol. 1, pp. 100–101).
13   See *International Statistical Classification of Diseases and Related Health Problems*, 10th rev. (Albany, 1992), F32.3.
14   From Dr Pauline Watson, in personal correspondence to Stephen W. Sykes, 2002.
15   *Letters*, vol. 1, p. 40.
16   *Letters*, vol. 1, p. 101.
17   Steele in a letter from 18 June, 1709, cited in Jenny Uglow, *Hogarth: A Life and a World* (London, 1997), p. 256.

18 This plate can be found in *Hogarth*, p. 256. These are the closing words of a poem by John Hoadly, which accompanied the print in *A Rake's Progress*, and cited in *Hogarth*, p. 257.

19 *Hogarth*, p. 258.

20 Available as *Olney Hymns in Three Books* (Olney, 1979).

21 *Poems*, vol. 1, pp. 174–75.

22 *Letters*, vol. 2, pp. 454–55.

23 In a letter to Joseph Hill, 12 November 1776, *Letters*, vol. 1, p. 265.

24 *Letters*, vol. 2, p. 385.

25 The text of which appears at http://www.igracemusic.com/gracemusic/hymn-writers/CowpersFuneral.htm.

26 See George Kelvin Ella, *William Cowper: Poet of Paradise* (Darlington), pp. 518–21.

27 In *Poems*, vol. 2, pp. 109–303.

28 To Lady Hesketh, 14–16 January, 1787, *Letters*, vol. 3, pp. 14–15.

29 'There is nothing but this, no Occupation within the Compass of my small Sphere, Poetry excepted, that can do much towards diverting that train of Melancholy thoughts, which when I am not thus employ'd, are for ever pouring themselves in upon me' (18 March 1781, to John Newton, *Letters*, vol. 1, p. 459).

30 'To Mary', *Poems*, vol. 3, p. 207.

31 *Letters*, vol. 1, p. 393.

32 Mary Tofts was the woman who had claimed, and was widely believed by fashionable medical men, to have given birth to rabbits in 1726.

33 Uglow, *Hogarth*, p. 653.

34 *Poems*, vol. 1, p. 325.

35 See M. C. Battestin, ed., *Joseph Andrews* (Oxford, 1967).

36 'Holy Willie's Prayer' did not appear in Burns' first compilations of poetry, namely the 1786 Kilmarnock and 1787 Edinburgh editions. It was, however, popular and circulated orally until it was published in a pamphlet in 1789, perhaps the version that was read by Cowper. See Thomas Crawford, *Burns: A Study of His Poems and Songs* (Edinburgh, 1960).

37 One William Fisher, an Ayrshire farmer who was elder of a kirk session which pursued a friend of Burns.

38 See R. Cecil, *The Works of Rev. John Newton* (Edinburgh, 1846).

39 *Olney Hymns* vol. 1, p. 64, stanza 1.

40 Stanza 6.

41 *The English Hymn* (Oxford, 1997), p. 290.

42 See *The Stricken Deer*, p. 84ff.

43 Vincent Newey, *Cowper's Poetry: A Critical Study and Reassessment* (Liverpool, 1982), p. 274, emphasis original.

44 *Letters*, vol. 1, p. 335.

45 *Letters*, vol. 1, p. 341.

46 *Letters*, vol. 1, p. 393.

47 *Letters*, vol. 1, p. 395.

48 See in the version of *The Book of Common Prayer*, Psalms 42, 46, 55, 61, 65, 68, 77, 78, 83, 88, 89, 93, 107, 124, 130, 139.

49 *Cowper's Poetry*, pp. 306–13, see particularly p. 312.

50 *Cowper's Poetry*, p. 275.

51 The very term, 'castaway', is itself from the Bible. St Paul makes clear to his church in Corinth that to be a decent apostle he has to be self-disciplined, 'lest that by any means, when I have preached to others, I myself should be a

castaway' (1 Cor 9:27). Cowper had earlier used the word in one of his hymns, entitled 'Welcome Cross':

> Did I meet no trials here,
> No chastisement by the way;
> Might I not, with reason, fear
> I should prove a cast-away (*Poetry*, 1. 176).

52 From 'The Castaway'.
53 See Stephen W. Sykes, 'Sacrifice and the Ideology of War', in *The Institution of War*, ed. Robert A. Hinde (Houndmills, 1991), pp. 87–98.

7

'Mad as a refuge from unbelief': Blake and the Sanity of Dissidence

David Fuller

'There are states in which all visionary men are accounted mad men.'[1] As a result of dissent from norms of his culture in poetry, visual art, and religion Blake was such a visionary: he was accounted 'mad'. His annotations of the phrenologist J. G. Spurzheim's *Observations on the Deranged Manifestations of the Mind, or Insanity* (1817) indicate one response.

> Cowper came to me and said, 'O, that I were insane always. I will never rest. Can you not make me truly insane? I will never rest till I am so. O, that in the bosom of God I was hid! You retain health, and yet are as mad as any of us all – over us all – mad as a refuge from unbelief, from Bacon, Newton, and Locke.' (E, 663)

In this visionary visitation 'madness' (so-called) is supreme evidence of sanity: what is here called 'mad' is, from a properly human perspective, sanity unacknowledged and disallowed – a way of evading the true madness of believing, for example, that spiritual realities have a determining material basis. That is what, for Blake, the Unholy Trinity of Bacon, Newton and Locke signify. There is an irony in Blake's invoking Cowper in this way. For Cowper madness was a terrible affliction. It drove him – as Blake's eccentricity and dissent never did – into a madhouse. He did not relish it, as Blake at times relished his supposed 'madness', as the index of a valuable alienation. In Blake's Spurzheim annotation 'mad' is used in two senses: non-metaphorical – the kind of affliction that sent Cowper into an asylum; and metaphorical, a negative term adopted with a positive charge – alienation from inert conventions and habits; an active opposition to materialist philosophies. To escape succumbing to the world view of Blake's Trinity of Error – Bacon, Newton, Locke – is to be 'hid in the bosom of God'.

Blake was alienated from the presuppositions of his own culture, but he knew that it was the culture, not him, that was parochial; that his view of the value of the supra-rational, however out of tune with his age, had grand antecedents. Both classical and biblical writers had ways of seeing madness in positive terms. In the *Phaedrus*, in the person of Stesichorus Socrates presents madness, 'provided it comes as the gift of heaven', as 'the channel by which we receive the greatest blessings: ... Madness comes from God, whereas sober sense is merely human'. Socrates specifically gives among his examples the poet, possessed by the Muses.[2] He gives a similar account of inspiration in the *Ion* (sections 535–6). This positive vision of madness in Greek writing is paralleled in Roman writers.[3] Drawing together this classical tradition in his *Discoveries* Ben Jonson cites examples from Plato to Ovid.[4] Christian tradition suggested a comparable view. The symbolic actions of the prophets, taken over by God who speaks through them, gain some of their force from being extravagantly at odds with common sense. Speaking in tongues St Paul specifically calls 'mad' from the perspective of the unbeliever (1 Corinthians, 14.23). Similarly indicative is his revaluative inversion of wisdom and folly: 'the wisdom of this world is foolishness with God' (1 Corinthians, 3.19). Madness in Elizabethan drama, and above all in Shakespeare, is associated with dissident insight – the madness of Hamlet, and still more the madness of King Lear: alienation from conventional understanding prompts depths of perception to which habit and custom have previously made the character blind. The Augustan eighteenth century moved away from this. In beginning to recover the classical-biblical-Shakespearean sense of madness as connected with genius, inspiration, freedom from convention – an ability to respond adequately to what is valuable in what is extraordinary – Blake is in tune with a decisive shift in sensibility.

The first intimations of this shift can be found in his earliest work, the youthful *Poetical Sketches* (1783), with its 'Mad Song' (*SPP*, 48–9).

> The wild winds weep,
>   And the night is a-cold;
> Come hither, Sleep,
>   And my griefs enfold.
> But lo, the morning peeps
>   Over the eastern steeps,
> And the rustling birds of dawn
>   The earth do scorn.
>
> Lo, to the vault
>   Of pavèd heaven
> With sorrow fraught
>   My notes are driven;
> They strike the ear of night,
>   Make weep the eyes of day;
> They make mad the roaring winds,
>   And with tempests play.

Like a fiend in a cloud
With howling woe,
After night I do crowd,
And with night will go;
I turn my back to the east,
From whence comforts have increased,
For light doth seize my brain
With frantic pain.

Blake owned a copy of Bishop Percy's *Reliques of Ancient English Poetry* (1765). The collection, part of a later eighteenth-century vogue for the primitive, included six mad songs, and Percy noted in a preface to them how much more common mad songs were in English than in other European literatures. Writing in the 1770s the teenage Blake was in part native and in the fashion. But Blake's poem is also unusual. It is sympathetic to the mad speaker, which not all mad poems are. And Blake's reader is not told why the speaker is mad. Most of Percy's songs are about love-madness. In Blake's poem the speaker is radically or metaphysically mad – one whose kinship with night, tempests, roaring and howling is not, as a forsaken lover's would be, contingent. In the final stanza he seeks with demonic pleasure an environment that will allow madness scope. He is driven to this apparently perverse indulgence by flight from the alternative: paradoxically, comfort is painful. A poem that begins (conventionally) with the sufferings of madness ends (unusually) with the sufferings of trying not to be mad, if mad you are. It is a first intimation of an unusual way of seeing the subject.

This is consistent with the way Blake treats other outcast or dissident figures, as in the later lyric, 'Mary' (*SPP*, 280–82). Mary is exceptional (in beauty, but the issue is exceptionality in any form), but admiring recognition of this turns to envy. Mary responds to antagonism by trying to conceal what marks her out: as a result she is treated as mad, caught in a double-bind of alienation – damned both for being, and for trying not to be unusual. That Mary was seen by Blake as an alter-ego is implied by Blake's use of two lines from the lyric as the opening of a poem about himself that describes the Mary syndrome – failing to deal successfully with being unusual by dealing negatively with what makes him so.

O, why was I born with a different face?
Why was I not born like the rest of my race?
When I look each one starts; when I speak I offend.
Then I'm silent and passive, and lose every friend.

Then my verse I dishonour, my pictures despise,
My person degrade, and my temper chastise,

And the pen is my terror, the pencil my shame;
All my talents I bury, and dead is my fame.

I am either too low or too highly prized;
When elate I am envied, when meek I'm despised.

(E, 733)

The poem follows Blake's account of an altercation with a soldier that led to his being tried on a charge of sedition: it was written at a time when he had more than his usual reasons for feeling an outsider. He adopts or articulates a persona of the alienated outcast whose wisdom is at odds with received practice, and whose characteristic gestures, signifying identity and purpose, are 'mad' – that is, abnormal or disallowed in terms of accepted behaviour. It recalls Blake's first experiment with illuminated printing, *All Religions Are One* (1788), with its epigraph 'the voice of one crying in the wilderness'. Blake is John the Baptist, a character of ostentatious weirdness, who prepares the way of the Messiah. Blake prepares the way for himself.

Later, through the figure of Los, the personification of the imaginative powers, Blake shows how such alienation is basic to artistic creativity. We can see Blake working towards this figure in his presentation of the dissident visionaries, Isaiah and Ezekiel, in *The Marriage of Heaven and Hell*.

The prophets Isaiah and Ezekiel dined with me, and I asked them how they dared so roundly to assert that God spake to them; and whether they did not think at the time that they would be misunderstood, and so be the cause of imposition.

Isaiah answered, 'I saw no God, nor heard any in a finite organical perception; but my senses discovered the infinite in everything, and as I was then persuaded, and remain confirmed, that the voice of honest indignation is the voice of God, I cared not for consequences but wrote.'

Then I asked, 'Does a firm persuasion that a thing is so, make it so?'

He replied, 'All poets believe that it does, and in ages of imagination this firm persuasion removed mountains; but many are not capable of a firm persuasion of anything.' ...

I also asked Isaiah what made him go naked and barefoot three years. He answered, 'The same that made our friend Diogenes the Grecian.'

I then asked Ezekiel why he ate dung, and lay so long on his right and left side. He answered, 'The desire of raising other men into a perception of the infinite. This the North American tribes practise; and is he honest who resists his genius or conscience only for the sake of present ease or gratification?'

(*The Marriage of Heaven and Hell*, plates 12–13; SPP, 134–6)

Basic here is Blake's irony and its significance. In what is at first presented unequivocally as visionary experience one of the visitor-visionaries is asked about the nature of visions. He affirms, equally unequivocally, that the sense in which the visionary sees anything is entirely symbolic ('I saw no God, nor heard any ... but my senses discovered the infinite in everything'). This sophisticated teasing of any would-be literalist reader goes hand-in-hand – despite the usual Hebraic monotheist exclusivist claims to which Ezekiel refers – with a non-exclusivist religious stance. Isaiah compares himself with Diogenes (another dissident who engaged in weird symbolic actions); Ezekiel compares himself with 'the North American tribes'. As Blake's tractate has it, all religions are one. The teasing is accompanied by an appropriate comic tone. True as it may be fundamentally, Ezekiel takes striking short cuts when he gives his reason for 'eating' dung (itself an extravagantly elliptical representation of the biblical account), and for lying 390 days on his right side and forty days on his left: 'the desire of raising other men into a perception of the infinite'. This is writing brilliantly in control of tone, and precisely over areas – the nature of visionary experience, and the claims of religious truth – where any tendency to a breakdown of control is most likely to show itself. This is writing about what eighteenth-century sanity called madness – the claim to see visions – but the writing itself is quite the reverse of lunatic: it is ironic, comic, intelligent, poised.

Battling in a life-and-death struggle with a culture that he saw as deeply antagonistic to spiritual life, poised and ironic is not Blake's characteristic stance. When Isaiah sneers that 'many people are not capable of a firm persuasion of anything' he adumbrates an alternative to the poised, ironic mode.

Infected, mad, [Los] danced on his mountains, high, and dark as heaven.
Now fixed into one steadfast bulk, his features stonify.
From his mouth curses, and from his eyes sparks of blighting;
Beside the anvil cold, he danced.

(The Four Zoas, 57.1–4; E, 338)

Los is not poised, and Blake's account reflects his subject. Los has here reached a significant stage in his fall from eternal into temporal being. The last potentially redemptive faculty of Blake's archetypal human psyche, Los has just completed the creation in the fallen world of his complementary anti-type, Urizen. The keynote of this seven-day de-creation is that 'bones of solidness froze over all [Urizen's] nerves of joy' (*The Four Zoas*, 54.14; E, 336). In order to cope with the conditions of temporal existence, what was fluxile and responsive becomes fixed and insensible; and Los takes on the rigidity of the being he has 'created': 'terrified at the shapes / Enslaved humanity put on, he became what he beheld. / He became what he was doing. He was himself transformed' (*The Four Zoas*, 56.21–3; E, 338). In Blake eternal beings can at will contract or expand infinite senses, inlets of awareness and knowledge. The ability marks a difference between living and merely existing. Los's senses – potential inlets of this higher state of being – in his fall become 'unexpansive'. Fresh to this state of conformity to the conditions of temporal life, consciousness of what he has lost makes Los rage against his condition. His madness is the rage of oppressed sanity.

In *Milton* the mythical Los, archetype of the creative faculty, is replaced by the historical John Milton, poet. Like Los, in grappling with the fallen world Milton too 'became what he beheld'. In *Milton* he returns to earth to recant his errors, particularly his misrepresentation of Christianity in *Paradise Lost*, where it is associated with classical epic and so (in Blake's view) with an unchristian heroic militarism. By struggling to rehumanise the faculty fixed by Los into an unexpansive fallen form (Urizen), and by reuniting with his alienated feminine aspects, Milton comes to understand how to transcend the oppressions that drove Los to madness.

> To bathe in the waters of life, to wash off the not-human ...
> To cast aside from poetry all that is not inspiration,
> That it no longer shall dare to mock with the aspersion of madness
> Cast on the inspired by the tame high finisher of paltry blots
> Indefinite, or paltry rhymes, or paltry harmonies ...
> To cast off the idiot questioner, who is always questioning
> But never capable of answering, who sits with a sly grin
> Silent plotting when to question, like a thief in a cave,
> Who publishes doubt and calls it knowledge, whose science is despair,
> Whose pretence to knowledge is envy, whose whole science is
> To destroy the wisdom of ages to gratify ravenous envy ...
> These are the destroyers of Jerusalem, these are the murderers
> Of Jesus, who deny the faith and mock at eternal life.

(Milton, plate 43.1–22; SPP, 301–2)

Milton here delivers one of the great summary doctrinal statements in Blake's later poetry on the intellectual, spiritual and creative life. He addresses, as Blake sees them, the problems all individuals face in discovering, developing and preserving their creativity. But from the point of view denounced, the manner of denunciation demonstrates the objections to its substance. While from a point of view convinced of prophetic insight Milton embodies an exhilarating exuberance of conviction, to a would-be dispassionate reasoner (to Blake a sly questioner) Milton displays the lunatic's monocular vision. To a Socratic debater the repetition of key terms and structures of prophetic discourse epitomises the obsessive:

Milton is mad. Whatever sympathy a reader feels with the terms of the denunciation, many will surely also harbour some sense that anyone who denounces with such unequivocal conviction might well cast a reasonable sceptic in the role of idiot questioner and denouncee. The rhetoric is the character's, not the author's; but the implications of its mode – its stance of no negotiation with alternative views – is endorsed by the parallel implications of Blake's formal strategies in *Milton*. Radically at odds (for this period) with any reader's formal expectations of epic, *Milton*'s non-narrative embodiment of the claim that all the elements of a poem's conception take place 'in a moment' similarly makes no negotiation with conventional formal expectations: these are simply cast aside. The reader's experience is of being confronted with sense-making demands uncompromisingly on the poet's terms. The most common initial response is incomprehension – the response of the poet Robert Southey when Blake showed him *Jerusalem*, which Southey judged 'a perfectly mad poem': 'Oxford Street is in Jerusalem', he jibed, as evidence of its madness. In fact *Jerusalem*, personification of the visionary city of Revelation, is in Oxford Street – as well she might be in a symbolic poem about the spiritual state of England. Nevertheless, Southey 'held [Blake] for a decided madman'.[5]

The movement shown through Los (in *The Four Zoas* and in *Jerusalem*) towards mental and emotional derangement is a constant subject of Blake's work. His poetry is full of characters who are spiritually sick, or are driven to despair or extreme states of scarcely controllable mental suffering, by infection from the surrounding culture, which corrupts love, art, religion, intellectual and spiritual life. Blake's fundamental myth of four *zoas* ('living creatures', from the Greek of Revelation, 4.6) is used to symbolise this disharmony within the individual psyche. There is always a thin line between extreme stress arising from intellectual and spiritual malaise and a final collapse into the deranged. When the zoas battle against one another one thing imaged is an extreme of mental torment which, as these internecine struggles reach points of crisis, shades into madness. 'There they take up / The articulations of a man's soul, and laughing throw it down / Into the frame; then knock it out upon the plank, and souls are baked / In bricks to build the pyramids' (*Jerusalem*, 31.9–12; *SPP*, 319). The biblical archetype of oppression shows the pattern of all societies: individuality is suppressed in favour of performing one's role in the structure. The result is that 'all the tendernesses of the soul [are] cast forth as filth and mire' (*Jerusalem*, 31.21; *SPP*, 319). Inhuman values act like funnels down which the mind is dragged. Codes that place barriers between love and sexual expression show a characteristic cycle of corruption. Free play of intellect narrows into obsession with the love that is denied; love denied narrows to sexual desire; frustrated desire creates an inward chaos of feeling that is channelled outwards into love's anti-type, violence. As Blake images it, once the roots of Albion's tree – a corrupt, proliferating growth of the banyan type, the branches of which also put down roots – have entered the soul, one form of spiritual sickness leads inevitably to another.

Los's agon (Plate 1) is that of the creative aspects of the personality. It is expected to be the reader's. It draws on Blake's own struggles to create and to find an audience. Blake is also present in his work in his own person, recording his personal witness in the manner of an Old Testament prophet, and, like a self-conscious modern, recording his struggle to give his perceptions form. There is a constant sense in his later work of how difficult and painful the search for understanding and expression can be. In this context even the occasional dogmatisms convey not Olympian, above-the-struggle certainty but rather assertive desperation. But though Los is 'the labourer of ages in the valleys of despair' (*Jerusalem*, 83.53; E, 242), despair can be kept at bay. There are also struggles to re-humanise. Sources of affection and inspiration can be protected: they can be preserved in and recovered through art. Music, poetry and painting are 'powers of conversing with paradise' ('A Vision of the Last Judgement'; E, 559) – being kept aware of a world other than the mundane. Art not only images the struggle to retain sanity: it also ministers to the sick.

Blake's most notable graphic work on madness is his colour print 'Nebuchadnezzar' (Plate 2).[6] It carries a meaning quite different from that imaged by the trials of Los. One of a series of twelve works conceived (and perhaps executed) in 1795, at the end of Blake's first period of engraving illuminated poetry, its subject is biblical, from the book of Daniel. Nebuchadnezzar, ruler of Babylon, dreams of a great and flourishing tree which is cut down by order from heaven, but with a stump and roots remaining. The king's soothsayers are not able to interpret the dream. It is interpreted by the Hebrew prophet, Daniel: the tree is a symbol of Nebuchadnezzar, its cutting down a punishment for sin. Daniel advises righteousness, particularly showing mercy to the poor. Nebuchadnezzar responds by trusting in his power.

> While the word was in the king's mouth, there fell a voice from heaven, saying, O king Nebuchadnezzar, to thee it is spoken; the kingdom is departed from thee. And they shall drive thee from men, and thy dwelling shall be with the beasts of the field: they shall make thee to eat grass as oxen, and seven times shall pass over thee, until thou know that the most High ruleth in the kingdom of men, and giveth it to whomsoever he will. The same hour was the thing fulfilled upon Nebuchadnezzar: and he was driven from men, and did eat grass as oxen, and his body was wet with the dew of heaven, till his hairs were grown like eagles' feathers, and his nails like birds' claws. (4.31–3; Authorized Version).

Thereafter Nebuchadnezzar acknowledges God's power and recovers his reason. The text concludes: 'those that walk in pride [God] is able to abase'.

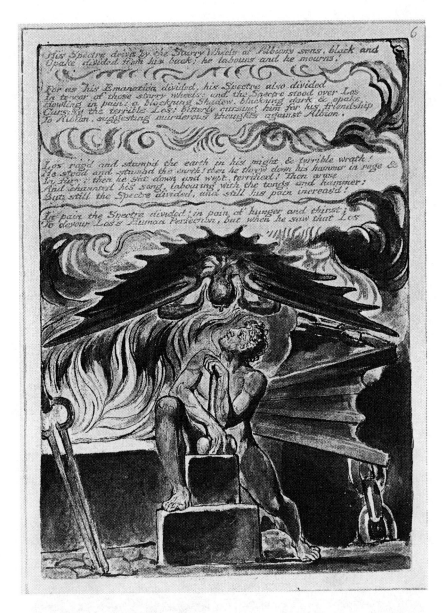

Plate 1. *Jerusalem*; relief etching, printed in orange, with pen and watercolour; 22.2
by 16.2 cms. Yale Centre for British Art, Paul Mellon Collection.

Los, whose creative work leads Blake to depict him as a blacksmith, is shown at his
forge, with fire, bellows, hammer, anvil and tongs. He looks up at his bat-winged
Spectre – the personification of his paranoia, who attempts to undermine his work
by encouraging hatred, doubt and fear.

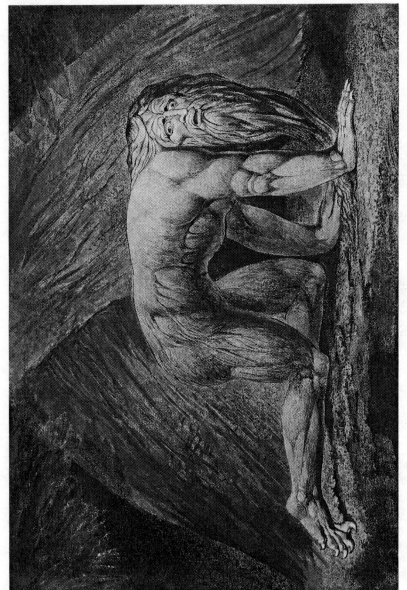

Plate 2. 'Nebuchadnezzar'. Colour Print, finished in ink and watercolour, 44.6 by 62 cms. Tate Gallery, London.

Blake probably thought of his twelve colour prints as a set. Though they are various in subject (based on the Bible, Milton, Shakespeare, and Blake's own myth), the common medium and size, the 1795 date inscribed on several, some apparent pairings, and the fact that a full set was bought by Blake's patron, Thomas Butts, suggest that they belong together. Among the visually thematic pairs 'Nebuchadnezzar' belongs with 'Newton'. 'Newton' is based on an illustration of Blake's early tractate, *There is No Natural Religion*, where it has the text, 'He who sees the infinite in all things, sees God. He who sees the ratio only, sees himself only' (E, 3). Staring down at his mathematical diagrams, Newton fails to perceive the divine. 'Nebuchadnezzar' is based on a design in *The Marriage of Heaven and Hell*, which has the caption, 'One law for the lion and ox is oppression' (plate 24; SPP, 145). This associates Nebuchadnezzar with the tyrannous Urizen's orders that all conform to a single standard, culminating in his command of 'one King, one God, one Law' (*The Book of Urizen*, 4.40; SPP, 215). The *Marriage* design's crown (absent from the colour print), along with the revolutionary and contemporary text that immediately follows, 'A Song of Liberty', may, in the 1790s, suggest a reference to contemporary politics – not only to the bestial nature of any tyrant, but specifically to the madness of George III. Blake was not always sympathetic to the mentally deranged. Nebuchadnezzar and Newton are the reverse of characters such as Los, driven mad by his attempt 'to [keep] the divine vision in time of trouble' (*Jerusalem*, 95.20; E, 255). Like Cowper in the visitation recorded in Blake's Spurzheim, Los is driven to madness by resisting materialism. Nebuchadnezzar is mad as a result of his failure to resist.

Los the artist, wrestling with the corruptions of Blake's society, is also Los the guardian. Searching through London with his globe of fire, he sees the poor and the oppressed, including the inmates of Bedlam.

[Los] came down from Highgate through Hackney and Holloway towards London,
Till he came to old Stratford, and thence to Stepney and the Isle
Of Leutha's Dogs, thence through the narrows of the river's side,
And saw every minute particular, the jewels of Albion, running down
The kennels of the streets and lanes as if they were abhorred. ...
And all the tendernesses of the soul cast forth as filth and mire
Among the winding places of deep contemplation intricate
To where the Tower of London frowned dreadful over Jerusalem, ...
... thence to Bethlehem, where was builded
Dens of despair in the house of bread. Enquiring in vain
Of stones and rocks he took his way, for human form was none.

(*Jerusalem*, plate 31[45].14–27; SPP, 319–20)

Though Blake did not finish *Jerusalem* until about 1820 and Bedlam moved in 1815, he is apparently thinking of Los here going to the old hospital.[7] All the other locations in Los's journey are north of the Thames: he comes from the villages north of London to the river's north bank, reaching Bedlam immediately after leaving the Tower – that is, the old Bedlam, in Moorfields. The most notable public concern about mistreatment in the hospital, registered in the report of a Parliamentary Select Committee of 1815, comes too late to have informed the passage. But the conditions in which people were kept were well-known before the formal investigation of 1814–15: that was why the investigation came about. The report shows that inmates were kept several to a room, naked except for a blanket gown, chained up or in yet more drastically restraining forms of fetters, with no distinction between the completely raving and those who in any modern sense would not be seen as 'mad' at all. Staff were little checked, so that violence and sexual abuse were endemic. Blake points up the etymology of the hospital's name, Bethlehem ('house of bread'), to enforce the irony of how the supposed place of care has become a 'den of despair'. The Tower and Bedlam have the same significance: to Los's prophetic sight both are indices of his culture's corruptions. If a civilisation can be judged by its prisons, so too can it be judged by its madhouses – which in this period were more-or-less forms of prison. Los chooses Bedlam, along with the Tower, as a place indicative of the nature of his society. As so often with Blake, the historically specific has a larger meaning. The wider implications of Blake's treatment are Foucaultesque: madhouses are created by intellectual conventions and social conditions that should not be taken at their self-evaluation.

Bedlam was the most famous madhouse of Blake's day. The asylum inmate of most concern to him was William Cowper. Blake was closely involved in the writing of the first biography of the poet. Its author, William Hayley, worked on the biography over exactly the period during which Blake lived alongside him under his patronage, from 1800 to 1803. Blake's role was to engrave the biography's illustrations, and it was in part to do this that he moved to live near Hayley, on the Sussex coast at Felpham. Hayley's biography of Cowper was therefore a principal ground of his patronage of Blake, and Hayley told Cowper's cousin, his principal associate in the project, Lady Harriet Hesketh, that Blake worked 'daily by my side on the intended decorations'.[8]

Hayley is explicit in the biography about drawing a veil over Cowper's mental afflictions.[9] He censored Cowper's letters to suit the views of Lady Hesketh, who wished to protect her cousin's posthumous reputation by minimising reference to his depressions and breakdowns. The biography gives no account of Cowper's confinements in a private asylum and attempts at suicide, and no explanation of the religious aspect of his depressions – his Calvinist conviction that he was among the reprobate, doomed to damnation. Working so closely with Hayley, Blake undoubtedly knew more about all this than the biography reveals. He may even have been drawn into the process of censorship. Lady Hesketh strongly disliked the portrait of Cowper by Romney that was to be engraved for the frontispiece: it conveyed too strongly the poet's 'distracted … look'. She was very much pleased when she found Blake's engraving had 'softened' the original and had 'an effect totally differently from that' of the portrait.[10] Her cousin no longer looked mad.

Blake rejected Cowper's theology, but he felt an affinity with him both as a poet and for the intensity of his religious experience. He also sensed (correctly) that Hayley saw the two poets in similar terms. In defending Blake from criticisms of the Cowper plates, Hayley commented on his 'dangerously acute' sensibility and 'excesses of feeling', and described Blake as like Cowper, 'of whom he often reminds me by little touches of nervous infirmity when his mind is darkened with any unpleasant apprehension'.[11] It was a comparison he often repeated, seeing particularly a kinship between the two poets in mental affliction.[12] Blake too felt a kinship with Cowper, but of a quite different kind. It was a kinship in what he supposed had been the manner of Hayley's friendship to the dead poet, paralleled by what, by 1803, he saw as Hayley's patronising manner to him, particularly Hayley's doubts about what Blake understood as 'inspiration'.

Blake's Notebook quatrains about Cowper also indicate that he saw some analogy (though as far as Hayley's treatment of Cowper goes this seems unjustified) between how Hayley failed in his supposed friendship to each of them, perhaps unconsciously: in Blake's view Hayley's conventional nature made him radically incapable of conceiving of life in the terms in which Blake saw it – and, Blake supposes, Cowper saw it too.

> William Cowper Esqre
>
> For this is being a friend just in the nick,
> Not when he's well, but waiting till he's sick.
> He calls you to his help; be you not moved,
> Until by being sick his wants are proved.
>
> You see him spend his soul in prophecy:
> Do you believe it a confounded lie,
> Till some bookseller and the public fame
> Proves there is truth in his extravagant claim;
>
> For 'tis atrocious in a friend you love
> To tell you anything that he can't prove,
> And 'tis most wicked in a Christian nation
> For any man to pretend to inspiration.
>
> (E, 507)

To a certain kind of prosaic nature, the poem implies, the whole claim to a special mode of consciousness ('inspiration') is a falsehood, or is at least misunderstood by more ordinary natures, and perhaps a source of antagonism from them. As in 'Mary', the exceptional ('mad' in the metaphorical sense) generates antagonisms that lead to alienation and a madness which, like Cowper's, is entirely non-metaphorical.

Blake attempted to embody what he saw as the fundamental issues of his conflict with Hayley in *Milton*. In the open section of the work – a song sung by an inspired Bard – Blake uses the Calvinist scheme of election and reprobation, but inverts the categories. Satan, of the elect, is self-righteous: he is an accuser of sin and opponent of imagination, at the farthest remove from the truly human and therefore (on Blake's view) the divine. His opponent, Palamabron, is of the reprobate: his qualities are unselfish love and imaginative freedom, both of which suffer under the self-righteous elect. Palamabron is driven to madness by Satan's incomprehension and unconscious tyranny, 'Seeming a brother, being a tyrant, even thinking himself a brother / While he is murdering the just' (*Milton*, 7.16–48 [22–3]; E, 100–101). In this conflict qualities endorsed as virtues by the surrounding culture are subjected to a scrutiny that gradually forces their true nature to reveal itself. They appear as covert egotism, an unconscious hypocrisy whose real desire is to impose on those whose creative openness to the real nature of existence, by giving them more to struggle with, makes them vulnerable to victimisation. The justice or otherwise of this to the historical William Hayley in his dealings with Cowper and Blake is beyond recovery. As a myth it is powerfully applicable to corruptions in the care of those deemed mentally ill whose difficulties and alienation are the result of a human fulness that cannot accept conventional ways of seeing and valuing.

Hayley represented generally accepted standards of taste for the time in poetry and painting, in both of which he was actively interested, as a successful poet and man of letters, and as an acknowledged connoisseur in fine art. He associated Cowper's genuine mental illness with Blake's uncompromising realisation of his own creativity, while such evidence as there is suggests that Blake probably saw Cowper's depressions as manifestations of creativity blocked or misunderstood. He was 'mad as a refuge from unbelief'. Blake may have had particular reasons for having Cowper in mind again when he read Spurzheim in about 1817. Cowper's own memoir, *Adelphi*, which treats his depressions, confinements and attempted suicide much more frankly than Hayley's *Life* had done, was published in 1816, and gave rise to a debate in the periodical press about the relation of Cowper's religious views to his insanity – whether his religion should be blamed for his depressions, or his depressions understood as only alleviated by his faith. Either way, poetry, madness, and religion were understood as the interrelated elements of his condition. Hayley understood Blake as like

Cowper, and both as mad. Blake understood himself as like Cowper, and both as creative beyond what ordinary sanity could understand.

Hayley was far from the only one of Blake's contemporaries to think of him as mad. It is a recurrent theme in contemporary comments on Blake and his work, both public and private. Most recent commentary has tended to imply that consideration of this is superseded, that it is an unreal issue which arose only because of conditions in Blake's culture, not because of things about Blake himself or his work.[13] But though the imputation of madness enraged Blake, he also appears at times to have encouraged it. In any case, the reception history of a writer, as of an individual work, is permanently part of his or her potential meaning. As Blake's devils put it: 'Everything possible to be believed is an image of truth' (*The Marriage of Heaven and Hell*, plate 8; *SPP*, 132). The point is to interpret: truth may be believed in images that are highly oblique.

We can see Blake apparently encouraging an imputation of literal belief in spiritual presences, of a kind that he must have recognised might be seen as verging on the insane, in his drawings of visionary portrait heads for the painter John Varley. It has been argued that these visionary heads reflect Blake's interest in contemporary medical psychology, in that they were influenced by his knowledge of phrenology – the pseudo-science of mental faculties supposed to be located in various parts of the skull and investigable by observing bumps on the head.[14] They may also indicate a puckish sense of humour. The accounts of the drawing sessions apparently show Blake taking – or affecting to take – the presence of his supposed sitters quite literally. Herod, Mohammed, the man who built the pyramids, the task-master Moses slew in Egypt, the ghost of a flea: these and many others came to Blake's rooms to sit for their portraits. Questions about whether Blake understood such visionary visits as literal or figurative feature regularly in discussions of his supposed 'madness' in early biographies.[15] It is not now possible to reconstruct what actually happened in the Varley drawing sessions, but it seems more than possible that Blake was having some innocent fun at the expense of the too easy credulity of friends. One must either explain the drawings in some such terms, or suppose that Blake had wholly abandoned the view of visionary experience offered in the more calculated effects of writing in *The Marriage of Heaven and Hell* where he teasingly calls to witness the authority of Isaiah and Ezekiel. Either way, while Blake seems to have been at least ready to play to the hilt and beyond the role of the Romantic Artist who drinks the milk of Paradise with a facility denied to ordinary mortals, none of the anecdotes about him seeing and conversing with spiritual visitants is incompatible with the position of Isaiah: 'I saw no [spirit], nor heard any, in a finite organical perception'.[16]

Doggerel verses scribbled in Blake's Notebook around 1810 show him reflecting on 'madness' (so-called) in a much more down-to-earth vein, having some knock-about fun with the issue to recuperate aesthetic criteria more suited to the appreciation of his own work. The lines treat a central element of his aesthetic – the importance of drawing to painting: he admired the clear outlines of Raphael and Michelangelo; he deplored what he thought of as the loss of form in indiscriminate colouring of Rubens and Rembrandt – 'shadows ... of a filthy brown, somewhat of the colour of excrement' (marginalia to Reynolds; E, 655). The verses veer about. The first couplet gives Blake's own view ('Painting ... exults in immortal thoughts', *A Descriptive Catalogue*, IV; E, 541), though filtered through the conceptions of his opponents (in calling his party mad; in his colloquial grammar: he is wild and untutored). He then adopts in caricature the view of his opponents (that drawing is an activity of hand; for Blake it is an activity of mind). His own view returns, with proper nouns as verbs for colloquial scorn (Fuseli is Blake's friend, the Swiss painter). Finally comes more advanced colloquialism (*OED*'s first recorded use of 'jaw' for 'lecture censoriously' is 1810), with 'mad' adopted again from his opponents ('madmen' in their view; in reality the true artists).

> All pictures that's painted with sense and with thought
> Are painted by madmen as sure as a groat,
> For the greater the fool, in the pencil more blessed,
> And when they are drunk they always paint best.
> They never can Raphael it, Fuseli it, nor Blake it;
> If they can't see an outline, pray how can they make it?
> When men will draw outlines begin you to jaw them.
> Madmen see outlines, and therefore they draw them.

> (E, 510)

This combative good humour shows Blake accepting 'mad' as the fool's reproach that is a kingly title.

Conversely, we see him enraged by the imputation of madness where it might be destructive of serious attention to his art. This happened most seriously in the reviews of his one solo exhibition in 1809. The reviewer was transformed into the epitome of the corruption of English culture in *Jerusalem*. Blake's annotations of Sir Joshua Reynolds' *Discourses* make it clear that he understood perfectly well that the fundamental battle is about the point of view from which judgements are made. As *The Marriage of Heaven and Hell* has it, 'the enjoyments of genius ... to angels look like ... insanity' (plate 6; *SPP*, 129). What some viewpoints see as mad, Blake sees as evidence of heightened perception, often more important insofar as it offends artistic or religious canons of what is orthodox. Blake is a writer like Flaubert, Wilde, Lawrence, Joyce, for whom offence to convention is a sign of spiritual, moral or aesthetic discovery. The value of the discovery may be in inverse proportion to the resistance it excites in conventional minds.

To Blake Reynolds was worse than conventional: 'this man was hired to depress Art' (E, 635). Blake's annotations of Reynolds' *Discourses* are, accordingly, combative in the highest degree.

Reynolds's opinion was that genius may be taught, and that all pretence to inspiration is a lie and a deceit to say the least of it. [If the inspiration is great why call it madness? *deleted*] For if it is a deceit the whole Bible is madness.

It is evident that Reynolds wished none but fools to be in the Arts, and in order to this [*sic*], he calls all others vague enthusiasts or madmen.

He who can be bound down is no genius. Genius cannot be bound. It may be rendered indignant and outrageous.

'Oppression makes the wise man mad.' Solomon [Ecclesiastes, 7.7].

(E, 642, 647, 658)

These expressively a-syntactic comments on 'Sir Joshua and his gang of cunning hired knaves' (E, 636) reveal Blake's angry recognition that the way in which Reynolds discounted supra-rational knowledge was to present it as irrational. But for Blake the biblical claim, particularly in the Prophets, that people can be vehicles of knowledge or wisdom when they are taken over by forces beyond themselves is a compelling form of witness that Reynolds' Neoclassical ideas about aesthetic knowledge as based on learned criteria are false. When Blake asked of the two most famous evangelists of eighteenth-century England, George Whitefield and John Wesley, 'were they prophets, / Or were they ... madmen?' (*Milton*, 22.61–2; E, 118), he was recognising that similar views underlie attacks on dissent in religion and in art. Both Reynolds' doubts about 'enthusiasm' and Blake's repudiatory marginalium arose from a common association between Protestant dissent and a Romantic critique of Neoclassical aesthetics – on the grounds that both Romanticism and Dissent appealed to potentially unregulated ideas of inspiration and an inner light. No ready-made criteria could therefore distinguish the Holy Spirit from the Devil in disguise, the poet from the poetaster, or illumination from lunacy. Accordingly, a usual way of dismissing Protestant dissent was to impugn it as madness. 'Enthusiasm' was a more ambivalent term for a range of negative perspectives. Like 'mad', it was therefore adopted by Blake as a positive. Los acts 'that enthusiasm and life may not cease' (*Jerusalem*, 9.31; E, 152); Blake opposes Reynolds with 'enthusiastic admiration ... the first principle of knowledge and its last' (E, 647); explaining himself to Hayley with a collection of recuperations, he is enthusiastic, mad and drunk: 'Excuse my enthusiasm, or rather madness, for I am really drunk with intellectual vision whenever I take a pencil or graver in my hand' (E, 757). 'Mad' is simply a crude weapon for the negative range of 'enthusiastic'.[17]

The more extreme term was frequently used of Blake by contemporary critics. As early as 1785 a reviewer of the Royal Academy's annual exhibition referred to his painting of Gray's Bard as 'mad'. In 1808 *The Anti-Jacobin's* review of his illustrations to Blair's *The Grave* took a similar line. After a negative discussion of the designs the reviewer turned to the dedicatory poem: 'Should he again essay to climb the Parnassian heights, his friends would do well to restrain his wanderings by the strait waistcoat.'[18] That Blake expected an attack somewhat in these terms on his exhibition of 1809 is clear from both his advertisement and his catalogue.[19] Expected though the terms of the attack apparently were, the review by Robert Hunt in *The Examiner* may have struck him as peculiarly savage.

> If ... the sane part of the people of England required fresh proof of the alarming increase of the effects of insanity, they will be too well convinced from its having lately spread into the hitherto sober region of Art. ... When the ebullitions of a distempered brain are mistaken for the sallies of genius by those whose works have exhibited the soundest thinking in art, the malady has indeed attained a pernicious height. ... Such is the case with the productions and admirers of William Blake, an unfortunate lunatic, whose personal inoffensiveness secures him from confinement. ... The praises ... bestowed last year on this unfortunate man's illustrations of Blair's *Grave* have, in feeding his vanity, stimulated him to publish his madness more largely.[20]

Blake's response, worked out in the privacy of his Notebook, was a mixture of cool irony and hearty repudiation.

> The painter hopes that his friends, Anytus, Melitus, and Lycon [the accusers of Socrates: to Blake, eternal types of *The Examiner's* editors, John, Leigh and Robert Hunt] will perceive that they are not now in ancient Greece, and though they can use the poison of calumny, the English public will be convinced that such a picture as this [Blake's 'Chaucer's Canterbury Pilgrims'] could never be painted by a madman ... as these bad men both print and publish by all the means in their power. ('Public Address'; E, 578)

The responses to Blake's work found in public comment are paralleled by those recorded in private remarks. Verses in the Notebook addressed to Blake's friend, the sculptor John Flaxman, indicate that Flaxman too had described Blake as mad (E, 507, 508). They show an anger similar to that of the Reynolds marginalia and the Public Address, but now in response not to a recognised opponent but to a friend and artistic associate. In a discussion of Blake as 'this insane man of genius', Wordsworth (who admired some of the *Songs* and copied them into his Commonplace book) is recorded by the diarist Henry Crabb Robinson as saying: 'There is no doubt this poor man was mad, but there is something in the madness of this man which interests me more than the sanity of Lord Byron and Walter Scott'.[21] Though it is clearly not what he meant in referring to Blake as 'mad', Wordsworth was not unsympathetic to Blake's fundamental argument about the kind of contest that is going on when the view that it is 'mad' is used to dismiss visionary writing. Wordsworth himself could view 'madness' as valuable dissidence, as in a notably Blakean passage of *The Prelude* on his own early experiences.

> Some called it madness: such, indeed, it was,
> If child-like fruitfulness in passing joy,
> If steady moods of thoughtfulness, matured
> To inspiration, sort with such a name;
> If prophesy be madness; if things viewed
> By poets in old time, and higher up
> By the first men, earth's first inhabitants,
> May in these tutored days no more be seen
> With undisordered sight: but leaving this
> It was no madness.

> (1805 text; 3.147–56)

The extended irony, culminating in 'tutored', is unusual, and indicates Wordsworth's hearty disdain for the judgement of the mediocre on the exceptional. The nexus of qualities is as in Blake: heightened consciousness (the uninhibited feelings of a child; the thoughtfulness of an adult), inspiration in art, prophecy in religion. Nevertheless, for Wordsworth Blake was mad in the plain sense.

This way of talking about Blake found its way straight into biography and criticism for almost a century after Blake's death. Allen Cunningham (1830), author of the most important biography before Gilchrist's; Edward FitzGerald (1833), translator of Omar Khayyám; James John Garth Wilkinson, the first to produce an edition of Blake's *Songs of Innocence and of Experience* in ordinary typography (1839); William Michael Rossetti, a principal figure in the Pre-Raphaelite Brotherhood, who edited the first substantial selection of Blake's poetry (1874); the conservative poet, Coventry Patmore, author of 'The Angel in the House' (on the role of women), for whom Blake's poetry was 'delirious rubbish', its author 'morally as well as intellectually mad', an epitome of nineteenth-century tendencies that needed keeping down (1889): all these and more – almost anyone who considered Blake's work, admirers and detractors – considered his sanity. When the *Journal of Psychological Medicine and Mental Pathology* ran a series on 'mad' artists, Blake duly made an appearance (1880). Even after the turn of the century the issue continued to be routinely discussed, albeit sometimes to be contradicted.[22] Even after Gilchrist's biography, in 1875, the painter and youthful friend of Blake's old age, Samuel Palmer, felt he needed to contradict an old and groundless report (1833) that Blake spent thirty years in a madhouse. His conclusion is striking: 'I remember William Blake, in the quiet consistency of his daily life, as one of the sanest, if not the most thoroughly sane man I have ever known.'[23]

***

Damit es Kunst giebt, damit es irgend ein äthetisches Thun und Schauen giebt, dazu ist eine physiologische Vorbedingung unumgänglich: der Rausch.
For art to exist, for any sort of aesthetic activity or perception to exist, a certain physiological precondition is indispensable: intoxication.

(Nietzsche, *Twilight of the Idols*, 'Expeditions of an Untimely Man', 8)

They will get it straight one day at the Sorbonne.
We shall return at twilight from the lecture
Pleased that the irrational is rational,
Until flicked by feeling.

(Wallace Stevens, *Notes Towards a Supreme Fiction*, III.x)

Unreasoning antagonism is not enough to account for the constant invocation of madness in relation to Blake – from many different shades of opinion, in public and in private; not always from opponents, not always from people disabled by lack of perception or vested interest. The constant invocation of madness points to real qualities in Blake's work. Now that Blake is a canonical figure in English poetry and visual art there is a value in refreshing the perception of these. How to describe these qualities is, of course, problematic: they might be described neutrally as a deep resistance to normalisation. Blake's complete association of form and content, for example, means that where there is novelty it is characteristic that it should be uncompromisingly, disorientatingly, in technique as well as subject-matter. But beyond this there is in Blake an unusual combination of qualities which mean that, even where he is most sympathetically understood, understanding is partial and in some interesting way skewed – achieved by a positive exclusion of what a different good light can make appear central. It is also a problem inherent in the study of Blake that reading techniques designed to enlighten, even when they are explicitly about the work's strangeness, have a normalising tendency that encounters resistance – because the weirdness of Blake's work is permanently part of what it means.

'It is impossible to say a great or noble thing', wrote Ben Jonson, 'unless the spirit is moved'. What is true for the writer is true also for the reader: it is impossible to *hear* a great or noble thing unless the spirit is moved. The reader as well as the poet needs to be in some sense 'mad'.

William Hazlitt remarked that age is spent finding out what one thought inarticulately in youth. It is grim to reflect that, for the reader who does not keep open channels to the madness of the Muses, increased ability of articulation may be accompanied by decreased intensity of perception: one might become more able to speak and have less to say. Rousseau may not be entirely right that 'it is impossible to think nobly if one thinks for a living' (*Confessions*, Book 8). He may not, either, be entirely wrong. There is probably some comparable truth about the practice of psychiatry: it is difficult to retain the human flexibility required to hear the deranged humanely if one listens for a living. That thinking is always conditioned by one's situation applies in particular ways if one's situation is that of a teacher. And beyond that, there is always some mismatch between the *understanding* of literature and the *study* of literature in institutions. This has to do in part with the acquisition of what passes for knowledge: in an educational context there is always a danger that information may stand in the place of understanding. Assessors have no speculative instruments with which to see if reading has (as Wordsworth puts it) rectified the feelings: they must settle for seeing whether or not some more testable form of comprehension has taken place. The mismatch between understanding that is worthwhile in human terms and understanding that is institutionally approved may have even more to do with the spirit in which knowledge is acquired – a conformity to fashionable suppositions, even (and sometimes most of all) within a nominal context of dissent and critique. This includes those forms of thought that a paradigm of knowledge derived from the sciences – knowledge as making progress – imposes on the arts. Institutions especially value this science-progress paradigm, though for reasons to do not with understanding but with funding. The templates of knowledge derived from the most economically powerful disciplines have built into them the assumption that one can study and teach literature as one can study and teach subjects in which objective information has a different role and status. Because the study and teaching of poetry, plays and novels is intertwined with issues of experience and value, the modes of knowledge, the structures within which thinking takes place, and the media of communication used are of the first importance. Those proposed or assumed by the contemporary university often do not fit well the understanding of literature. The contemporary equivalent of what Blake's visionary Cowper called 'unbelief', and Blake traced to Bacon, Newton and Locke, are the excesses of daylight, method, and order – in a word, 'sanity' – encouraged by bureaucratisation, mass-production and other characteristic pressures of contemporary literary education. These pressures squeeze out scope for relishing the weirdness of art and acknowledging the mysteries of understanding it.

Universities can further real knowledge of art, but one has often to work against the grain of institutions, which is increasingly towards knowledge regarded as uniform across disciplines. As a result, worthwhile study and teaching tends to take place in interstices rather than in formal situations. Current developments of education recognise the interstices, and the kind of knowledge implied by the interstitial, less and less. But the fit reader needs his or her responsive measure of the madness of the wild author. It is impossible adequately to *hear* a great or noble thing unless the spirit is moved. The art of William Blake is a paradigm for poetry, which is characteristically addressed to unusual states of consciousness. It is a paradigm not primarily in its content, nor in its mode, but in the flexibility required to hear the sanity beneath its surface weirdness.

Notes

1 *Laocoön*, in *William Blake: Selected Poetry and Prose*, ed. David Fuller (London, 2000), p. 361. All quotations from Blake are from this edition ('*SPP*'), except for material it does not include. This is quoted from *The Complete Poetry and Prose of William Blake*, ed. D. V. Erdman, with a commentary by Harold Bloom (New York, 1965, rev. edn, 1988), ('E'), but modernised on the principles described in *SPP* (pp. 18–26).

2 Plato, *Phaedrus*, trans. Walter Hamilton (Harmondsworth, 1975), pp. 46–8.

3 For example, and most famously, in Seneca: 'nullum magnum ingenium sine mixtura dementiae fuit' (there has been no great genius without a touch of insanity), *De tranquilitate animi*, xvii. 10.

4 *Ben Jonson*, ed. C. H. Herford and Percy and Evelyn Simpson, 11 vols (Oxford, 1925–52), vol. 8, p. 637.

5 G. E. Bentley Jr., *Blake Records* (Oxford, 1969), p. 229 (spelling and punctuation modernised).

6 Andrew M. Cooper, who provides copious information on contemporary cases and treatments of madness, suggests that some of the designs of Blake's illuminated books are based on the iconography of madness and its treatments, particularly 'Los howling' (the straitjacket), and Urizen 'in chains of the mind locked up' (fettered wrists and ankles): *The Book of Urizen*, plates 7 and 22; *SPP*, pp. 218, 232. 'Blake and Madness: The World Turned Inside Out', *ELH*, 57 (1990), pp. 585–642.

7 David Erdman argues for the building of 1815 (now the Imperial War Museum, near Blake's home of the 1790s in Lambeth), but this requires that Los cross the Thames and walk ten times the distance otherwise supposed: 'Lambeth and Bethlehem in Blake's *Jerusalem*', *Modern Philology*, 48 (1950–51), pp. 184–92.

8 Morton D. Paley assembles all the materials relevant to understanding Blake's involvement in 'Cowper as Blake's Spectre', *Eighteenth-Century Studies*, 1 (1968), pp. 236–52. There is also an account in Morchard Bishop, *Blake's Hayley* (London, 1951), chapters 17–19.

9 *The Life and Posthumous Writings of William Cowper*, 3 vols (London, 1803–4), vol. 1, p. 26.

10 *Blake Records*, p. 113.

11 *Blake Records*, pp. 105–6. Blake is also described as resembling 'our beloved bard [Cowper] in the tenderness of his heart and in the perilous powers of an imagination utterly unfit to take due care of himself'. As a whole the letter shows Hayley recognising what is unusual in Blake's work in positive terms.

12 'I have also every wish to befriend him [Blake] from a motive that, I know, our dear angelic Cowper would approve, because this poor man, with an admirable

quickness of apprehension and with uncommon powers of mind, has often appeared to me on the verge of insanity.' Letter to Lady Hesketh; *Blake Records*, p. 164.

13   But see G. E. Bentley Jr., *The Stranger from Paradise: A Biography of William Blake* (New Haven, CT, 2001), pp. 342 and 368–82.

14   Anne K. Mellor, 'Physiognomy, Phrenology, and Blake's Visionary Heads', in Robert N. Essick and Donald Pearce, eds, *Blake in his Time* (Bloomington, 1978).

15   For example, the discussion 'Mad or not Mad?' in the most important nineteenth-century biography, Alexander Gilchrist's (London, 1863; 2nd edn, 1880).

16   The most reliable anecdotes are those of Henry Crabb Robinson: *Blake Records*, pp. 535–49. Cf. the discussions of Seymour Kirkup: Bentley, *The Stranger from Paradise*, pp. 336–7.

17   See Susie I. Tucker, *Enthusiasm: A Study in Semantic Change* (Cambridge, 1972); Clement Hawes, *Mania and Literary Style: The Rhetoric of Enthusiasm from the Ranters to Christopher Smart* (Cambridge, 1996).

18   *Blake Records*, p. 208.

19   'Those who have been told that my works are but an unscientific and irregular eccentricity, a madman's scrawls, I demand of them to do me the justice to examine before they decide' (from the advertisement; E, pp. 527–8). 'This has hitherto been his lot [Blake's] – to get patronage for others and then to be left and neglected, and his work, which gained that patronage, cried down as eccentricity and madness' (*A Descriptive Catalogue*, III; E, pp. 537–8).

20   *Blake Records*, pp. 215–16. It may be indicative – or at least Blake may have thought it so – that from May to December 1808, *The Examiner* ran a series of seven essays, signed with Robert Hunt's symbol of the pointing hand, arguing 'the folly and danger of Methodism'.

21   *Blake Records*, p. 536. Cf. the Gothic novelist and book collector, William Beckford, on 'Mr. Blake, the mad draughtman's poetical compositions', which he compares to those of a thief who steals 'from the walls of Bedlam': *Blake Records*, p. 430.

22   Greville MacDonald, M. D., *The Sanity of William Blake* (London, 1908) (an expanded version of a lecture to the Ruskin Union); Joseph H. Wicksteed, 'The So-Called "Madness" of William Blake', *The Quest: A Quarterly Review*, 3 (1911), pp. 81–99. Wicksted wrote in response to G. K. Chesterton's *William Blake* (London, 1910), which contains an extensive discussion of Blake's 'madness'.

23   For Cunningham see *Blake Records*, pp. 476–507; for Wilkinson, Palmer, and *The Journal of Psychological Medicine and Mental Pathology* see G. E. Bentley Jr., *Blake Books* (Oxford, 1977), pp. 436, 881, 726; for FitzGerald see G. E. Bentley Jr., ed., *William Blake: The Critical Heritage* (London, 1975), p. 58. Rossetti's selection was published in the series the Aldine Poets; Patmore's essay in his *Principle in Art*. For other cases see Deborah Dorfman, *Blake in the Nineteenth Century: His Reputation as a Poet from Gilchrist to Yeats* (New Haven, 1969), pp. 34–44. On the claim Palmer refuted see Mona Wilson, *The Life of William Blake* (Oxford, 1927), appendix III.

8
'Why then Ile Fit You': Poetry and Madness from Wordsworth to Berryman

Michael O'Neill

According to Henry Nelson Coleridge, the poet's Boswell, Coleridge mused a few weeks before his death on the link between imagination and 'mania' in the course of clarifying a distinction between imagination and fancy:

> You may conceive the difference in kind between the fancy and the imagination in this way – that if the check of the senses and the reason were withdrawn, the first would become delirium, and the last mania. The fancy brings together images which have no connection natural or moral ... The imagination modifies images, and gives unity to variety; it sees all things in one.[1]

Seeing 'all things in one', the hallmark of the imaginative poet, is also, Coleridge contends, the characteristic of a person in the grip of mania. Arguably, his own opium-induced hallucinations gave him special insight into this condition. At any rate, in *Biographia Literaria*, illustrating Wordsworth's 'meditative pathos', Coleridge singles out two stanzas from 'The Mad Mother', concentrating on the last two lines of the first, where the mother sees even the action of the breeze in relation to her feelings: 'The breeze I see is in the tree! / It comes to cool my babe and me'. For Coleridge, here at his most luminously perceptive, the lines are 'expressive of that deranged state, in which from the increased sensibility the sufferer's attention is abruptly drawn off by every trifle, and in the same instant plucked back again by the one despotic thought, and bringing home with it, by the blending, fusing power of imagination and passion, the alien object to which it had been so abruptly diverted, no longer an alien but an ally and an inmate'.[2]

To speak of the mad mother making of the breeze 'an inmate', one might add, is a daring and affecting touch on Coleridge's part, flickeringly suggesting that the natural world is turned by the mother's 'despotic' imaginings into a consoling asylum full of 'inmates'. One might note, too, that Coleridge selects lines whose sounds threaten to collapse into echoes of the rhyme sound. It is striking, as we shall see, how often obsessive forms of rhyming or sound-patterning serve as a formal device that mimics 'monomania'. Often, in poems about madness, it is as though poets exploit the non-rational possibilities of sound-patterning to suggest fixations or disturbances of feeling. Certainly, the states dealt with in many of the poems discussed in this chapter fall under the heading 'mania', as Coleridge understands that term, that is, a 'deranged state' dominated by 'one despotic thought'. And yet these poems are fascinated by uniqueness rather than by classifications. In them madness eludes labels. Many of the poets in question are prepared to speak of 'madness', a term no longer in clinical or legal use, according to Peter Barham, since the Mental Health Act of 1959 'in which the "person of unsound mind" was replaced by the softer attribute of "mental disorder"'.[3] Yet they do so with a sense of the word as containing within itself an indefinable core. It may seem dangerous to generalise about poets as diverse in mode, and as separated by time and culture as Shelley and John Berryman. But both poets, like many of the greatest poets since 1800 who deal with madness, invite us to experience a kind of empathy with mental disorder. This empathy communicates through formal structures distinguished by their artistic order. Art and madness seem in this respect like one another's shadow selves in ways that this chapter – which seeks to be suggestive rather than comprehensive – will explore in relation to some poems written over the last two centuries.

Poets writing about madness may feel they are attempting to represent what is unrepresentable, or dangerous to represent. So we have Byron's puncturing of sentiment as he changes the subject after Haidee's affecting death in canto 4 of *Don Juan*: 'But let me change this theme, which grows too sad, / And lay this sheet of sorrows on the shelf; / I don't much like describing people mad, / For fear of seeming rather touched myself' (ll. 585–8).[4] The jokey tone, fending off what is feared, is meant to disconcert in a fashion characteristic of this poet. Almost one and a half centuries later, in 'A Mental Hospital Sitting-Room', Elizabeth Jennings moves from describing a reproduction of a painting by Utrillo in which a nun is 'climbing / Steps in Montmartre' to the line, 'It does not seem a time for lucid rhyming'. Lucid rhyming, however, is what she – and many poets writing about 'madness' – seem compelled to offer.[5] The effect in Jennings's poem is of a spell that wards off chaos, and yet a spell that pays homage to the dark enchantment of mental illness. 'Night Garden of the Asylum', by the same poet, finishes, 'We are in witchcraft, bedevilled', a line that rhymes with the last lines of the previous two stanzas; the patterning gives 'bedevilled' an effect of surprised, unmelodramatic closure.

In John Clare's 'I Am', rhyme is a marked formal feature that tells us we are reading a controlled utterance about experiential chaos. In this, the most gripping of Clare's asylum poems, the speaker clings to the first-person pronoun as though it were a spar from what he calls 'the vast shipwreck of my lifes esteems' (l. 10). Clare mimics God's self-definition, but his 'I am' comes from no burning bush. Rather, it issues from a sense of identity as torture. This is madness as unaccommodated but inexplicable selfhood, deserted by others, hopelessly nourished by 'woes': 'I am – yet what I am, none cares or knows; / My friends forsake me like a memory lost; – / I am the self-consumer of my woes' (ll. 1–3).[6] There is something bravely sardonic in this, for all its tragic extremeness. 'What am I?' asks Clare implicitly, then he responds with a reply that knows it is no answer: 'I am the self-consumer of my woes'. Self knows itself as it feeds on and is eaten up by suffering; form over-insists on its presence, as if to mimic the mind's futile yet speech-allowing stay against its own confusions. Clare's final stanza describes a longing for some simplified state, and 'mad poems' tend to be self-consuming artefacts, almost to burn up in the fires of a drive to order the chaotic. Alternatively, they may, as in lyrics from Thomas Lovell Beddoes's *Death's Jest-Book*, pitch themselves beyond any division between sanity and insanity, reason and unreason, and sing to us with a ghostly, grotesque beauty.

There is, in this tension between mental disorder and formal order, a heightened version of a tension between experience and artifice present in most poetry. Jacques Derrida, in 'Cogito and the History of Madness', his admiring critique of Michel Foucault's *Histoire de la folie*, comments that 'The misfortune of the mad, the interminable misfortune of their silence, is that their best spokesmen are those who betray them best; which is to say that when one attempts to convey their silence *itself*, one has already passed over to the side of the enemy, the side of order, even if one fights against order from within it, putting its origin into question'.[7] The antago-nism that Derrida finds between the unspeakableness of madness and the attempt to convey it turns, in many fine poems, into a tense intimacy. In Shelley's *Julian and Maddalo* the tussle between 'silence' and speech lies close to the heart of the poem's presentation of the Maniac, the character visited by the two friends and ideological opponents: Julian (an optimist, based on Shelley himself, but teased by the Preface as 'rather serious') and Maddalo (a pessimist, based on Byron, delightful in 'social life' but pos-sessed by 'an intense apprehension of the nothingness of human life').[8] The structure of the poem unfolds as a contest of interpretations. Julian admires the Venetian sunset as proving Italy to be a 'Paradise of exiles' (l. 57); Maddalo sees the brooding shape of a madhouse silhouetted against the sunset as an emblem of the human condition and tells Julian that, in his trust in the human will to make things better, he talks 'Utopia' (l. 179). They agree to visit a madman, whom Maddalo has helped; each friend sup-poses that the madman will be a 'case' that supports his view of life. They overhear the Maniac speak (he is not conscious of their presence), and they forego their debate: 'our argument was quite forgot' (l. 520), says Julian. The case-study has turned into a suffering person.

What Julian and Maddalo hear is a series of seemingly 'unconnected exclamations of ... agony', in Shelley's phrase in the Preface. The Maniac's mode of speech clashes with the urbanely conversational accents of the passages framing his soliloquy. Shelley makes use of ellipses to suggest his near-hysterical swervings of thought and feelings. These dots do not so much communicate dottiness as the will or need to hold at arm's length what keeps swinging back into view, some emotional violation experienced in a relationship with a woman. Gender issues cannot but suggest themselves here, and oblige us to recognise how many poems by male poets about madness express idealised longing for, or aggression towards, women. Often these feelings are worked through cathartically, so that the poem becomes more than the sum of its separate utterances. Potentially questionable or ugly emotions take us into difficult areas of feeling and result in a poetry that may profitably trouble the moral censor in us. Shelley's depiction is dramatic: that is, we are conscious that we have only the Maniac's word for various assertions. So, one paragraph ends with the self-martyring words, 'I live to show / How much men bear and die not!' (ll. 459–60), before passing, via a page-wide series of dots, into this, a slide into sickened recollection: 'Thou wilt tell / With the grimace of hate how horrible / It was to meet my love when thine grew less; / Thou wilt admire how I could e'er address / Such features to love's work' (ll. 460–5). The note of sexual hurt is strong and traumatic; in another passage (ll. 424–8), the Maniac recalls the woman wishing that he had castrated himself. We do not hear the woman's point of view; the Maniac's disturbed state is evident.

Shelley had been planning a work on the theme of the madness of Torquato Tasso, the Italian Renaissance poet, and traces of this subject remain in *Julian and Maddalo*, albeit transmuted. The listeners feel they have been in the presence of a poet, Julian saying, 'The colours of his mind seemed yet unworn; / For the wild language of his grief was high / Such as in measure were called poetry' (ll. 540–2). The 'colours' of the Maniac's mind, on this account, were not damaged. What has happened, according to Julian at first hearing, is that the Maniac is the victim of 'some dreadful ill / Wrought on him boldly, yet unspeakable, / By a dear friend' (ll. 525–7). Maddalo constructs from the Maniac's account a paradigm of the relationship between poetry and suffering: 'He said: "Most wretched men / Are cradled into poetry by wrong; / They learn in suffering what they teach in song"' (ll. 544–6) For all the dark irony of 'cradled' and the reversibility of the last line (which comes first – the teaching or the learning?), Maddalo offers an idealised view of the Maniac as poet-victim. Subsequently, without shifting his position exactly, Julian speaks of his wish to act as psychotherapist to the Maniac. In its patient respect for the 'caverns' of the mind, this is among the great accounts of psychological healing in literature: 'I imagined that if day by day / I watched him, and but seldom went away, / And studied all the beatings of his heart / With zeal, as men study some stubborn art / For their own good, and could by patience find / An entrance to the caverns of his mind, / I might reclaim him from his dark estate' (ll. 568–74). But the spun-out wish is ineffectual, just a fantasy. Julian, seeking relief from the 'deep tenderness' (l. 566) induced in him by the Maniac, leaves Venice the next morning, 'urged by my affairs' (l. 582). If Julian is ineffectual, the Maniac is ambiguous; he may have suffered some 'dreadful ill', but his interpretation of what went wrong with his relationship is subjective. Shelley dramatises his self-idealisation and self-pity without asking us to blame or praise, but rather to sympathise.

One lesson that the Maniac's soliloquy teaches is awareness of the gap between ideas about the human condition (such as those entertained by Julian, Maddalo and, indeed, the Maniac himself, who speaks of his 'creed', l. 359) and the thing itself. Even more fascinating is the struggle between the Maniac's desire to speak (and write) and his proto-Derridean sense of the vanity of language. His speech concludes with a triple rhyme that underscores his repeated longing for silence and death, and the poem is guarded against as well as open to interpretation. Madness retains its mystery. At the close of the poem, Maddalo's now grown-up daughter tells a chastened, older Julian how the Maniac and 'The Lady who had left him' (l. 599) reunited then parted again. This time, however, the reader is finally shut out from the poem, as though Shelley were enacting for us the impossibility of the very knowledge – of 'the beatings of [the] heart' – by a desire for which his poem has been impelled: 'I urged and questioned still, she told me how / All happened – but the cold world shall not know' (ll. 616–17).

Philippe Pinel (1745–1826) was a French physician who sought to treat the insane humanely, freeing most of his patients from the chains and irons which were the staple forms of restraint. His ideas were influential, none more so than the idea of *manie sans delire*, the notion, as Roy Porter explains it, of 'partial insanity (patients who were mad on one subject) in which the personality was warped but the understanding remained sound'.[9] Pinel's ideas were being disseminated at the dawn of some of the finest writings about madness in English poetry, and it is tempting to posit an epistemic connection between the idea of 'partial insanity' or monomania, and the new forms of monologue and monodrama. In a lecture of 1925 M. W. MacCallum argued that 'the object [of the dramatic monologue] is to give facts from within'.[10] How odd and potentially alienating these 'facts' can be is apparent from Browning's 'Porphyria's Lover'. At one stage (in 1836) the poem was published (with 'Johannes Agricola in Meditation') under the title 'Madhouse Cells', and one can see why. Here is the poem's climax: 'That moment she was mine, mine, fair, / Perfectly pure and good: I found / A thing to do, and all her hair /In one long yellow string I wound / Three times her little throat around, / And strangled her' (ll. 36–41).[11] Browning's metre – iambic octosyllabics – suits itself here to the speaker's murderously proprietorial attitude. He kills Porphyria to possess her completely, to keep her 'Perfectly pure and good'. The brutal decisiveness of thought and act ('I found / A thing to do') takes to an extreme the unspoken assumptions of corrupt forms of romantic love. The poem exposes as crazed any desire to convert the beloved into an idealised, unchanging object. The speaker is, in Robert Langbaum's words, 'undoubtedly mad', especially in his belief that Porphyria's 'darling one wish' (l. 57) (presumably to be with her lover) has been fulfilled and in his refusal wholly to accept that she is dead: 'her cheek once more / Blushed bright beneath my burning kiss' (ll. 47–8) is how he puts to himself the physiological effect of strangulation.

Yet we might wish to quarrel with Langbaum's assertion that 'Browning is relying upon an extraordinary complication of what still remains a rationally understandable motive'.[12] Langbaum underplays the element of emotional disorder and inexplicable urge to dominate in the poem. True, the speaker proceeds as though his behaviour were 'rationally understandable', but the gap between his assumption of rationality and our feelings of appalled fascination challenges understanding. In particular, we wonder about the workings of 'disordered subconscious urges' that Langbaum outlaws from discussion.[13] At the same time, these urges may express covert class tensions; the man appears to feel socially inferior to Porphyria and her 'vainer ties' (l. 24). Certainly, warning signals are communicated from the poem's opening, partly through the over-smooth rhymes and rhyming, and through the manner in which these formal features counterpoint the evidently unknowing projection of feeling on to the natural world: 'The rain set early in to-night, / The sullen wind was soon awake, / It tore the elm-tops down for spite / And did its best to vex the lake' (ll. 1–4). Sullenness and vexed spite may not be what the speaker thinks are at work in himself, but their latent presence is at least hinted at in a significant absence: after Porphyria has come in, warmed the place and taken off her dripping cloak and shawl, she 'sat down by my side / And called me' (ll. 14–15). The next phrase opens up an abyss: 'When no voice replied' (l. 15). The speaker has absented himself from his refusal to respond. Ultimately his proud response to her declaration of love will be to ensure that she is incapable of further response. The poem ends with the speaker looking elsewhere for conversation: 'And yet God has not said a word!' (l. 60), a line both terrified and triumphalist (as though latent guilt were being repressed and God's silence construed as divine approval). It could also be a challenge to God, such as is mounted in Browning's source, John Wilson's 'Gosschen's Diary', in which the speaker cries to God, 'Thou madest me a madman! ... I have done thy will ... am I a holy and commissioned priest, or am I an accused and infidel murderer?'[14] Browning lets his ambivalences group themselves more economically. But in tension with a progressivist view of madness as 'a logical and coherent extension of character', as the Longman editors gloss the position, the poem offers a vision of derangement bordering on evil.[15]

Tennsyon's *Maud*, originally titled *Maud or the Madness*, before being redubbed *Maud: a Monodrama* twenty years later in 1875, takes us back to Hamlet's tragically fraught and duplicitous form of insanity. Tennyson's son has this recollection: 'My father said, "This poem of *Maud or the Madness* is a little *Hamlet*, the history of a morbid, poetic soul, under the blighting influence of a recklessly speculative age. He is the heir of madness, an egoist with the makings of a cynic ... The peculiarity of this poem is that different phases of passion in one person take the place of different characters."'[16] As in many poems involving madness, the question of 'egoism' is to the fore, and yet we are less judgemental about than caught up in the speaker's 'different phases of passion'. After Maud has died, the speaker utters some of the most affecting lines that Tennyson ever wrote (part 2, section 4). The poem's hero, in this section, is haunted to the point of madness by an unnamed 'shadow'. At the climax of this section (stanzas 10–13), Maud, recalled 'glimmering' (stanza 11) like an ethereal ghost when alive, has now become, or her loss is symbolised by, the shadow that lures the speaker on, even as the speaker himself steals through the streets like a ghost. The last stanza reaps the reward of the beating away at the rhyme sound in 'street' which has run through the entire section, until flowering into lacerated blossom. The rhythms of the section are expressive of bipolar affective disorder, manic depression. In these lines from the section's final stanza, 'And I loathe the squares and streets, / And the faces that one meets, / Hearts with no leave for me' (stanza 13), Tennyson foreshadows the studied neuroses of T. S. Eliot's Prufrock, preparing a face to meet the faces that you meet. In *Prufrock*, however, Eliot weds terror to an ironic self-possession. In Tennyson's poem, the stanza in question shows how grief has generated a nightmarish state of fear, self-obsession and self-abasement that is, in Christopher Ricks's phrase, 'trembling on the brink of madness'.

Ricks points to 'the momentary stiffening in *one* ['the faces that one meets']' as possessing a 'pathetic fragility'.[17] That 'pathetic fragility' marries an insistence close to rage, communicating through the device of monorhyme and the assertiveness of 'I', as though the self were rebelling against, as much as submitting to, the shame-ridden anguish of stanza 10 in this section. The lines quoted above show how the final stanza of part 2, section 4 turns into a cry of hatred for others. But something else happens in the ensuing lines which conclude the section:

> Always I long to creep
> Into some still cavern deep,
> There to weep, and weep, and weep
> My whole soul out to thee.

Here hatred for and fear of others crosses with a feeling of being abandoned by 'Hearts with no love for me', and passes into a desire both to escape 'into some still cavern deep' and still to be heard by another, much as Shelley's Maniac both wishes to remain silent and desires to communicate. In the longing to 'weep, and weep, and weep / My whole soul out to thee', emotional mania pulses through the sounds. The suffering self wishes to gather itself up in that internally rhymed phrase 'whole soul' into a single word, the Logos of madness, before it exhales itself as an anguished gift to 'thee', rhyming tantalisingly with the shut-off 'me', 'thee' being the other beyond madness, looking down from 'among the blest' mentioned in the previous stanza.

In the next section of the poem (part 2, section 5), an unspoken rhyme makes itself felt as we pass from womb to tomb; the poem has crossed the border between sanity and madness. The longing to be in some 'still cavern deep' is here fulfilled in a 'deeply macabre' way, to borrow Ricks's phrase, since now the speaker imagines that he is 'dead, long dead, / Long dead!', buried in 'a shallow grave' 'Only a yard beneath the street'.[18] Throughout the poem, metre is the servant of madness; 'successive phases of passion' call forth resourceful variations. The mad scene retains rhyme and its lines scan, but there is no metrical norm. The lines enact, in their very move-ment, two things: a faltering, fluttering struggle to retain control, on the speaker's part, and his sense of the indifference to this struggle of 'the stream of passing feet, / Driving, hurrying, marrying, burying, / Clamour and rumble, and ringing, and clatter'. In the first line, the 'street' rhyme which has become insanity's motif is heard again; the series of gerunds in the second line repeats the world-weariness and loathing of modern society which the speaker – son of a melancholy suicide – has articulated in the poem's opening part. Madness is neighbour to an awareness of madness: 'to hear a dead man chatter / Is enough to drive one mad', the first stanza of this 'mad' section concludes, as though the speaker were not yet 'mad'. It is a ghoulish joke, since he has been driven 'mad', and yet the section is in tune with the social critique that runs through *Maud*, and brings to a head the poem's suggestion that madness embodies a legitimate protest against a society whose idea of sanity is 'lust of gain, in the spirit of Cain' (part 1, section 1, stanza 6). That is not to say that we accept uncritically the speaker's critique of society; but the descent into madness at the loss of Maud allows him to hit an authentic rock-bottom of despair. As a result, we wonder whether his supposed cure – the redemption he apparently under-goes in the third part when he goes off to fight in the Crimea to 'embrace the purpose of God, and the doom assigned' (stanza 5) – really is a cure. Is madness sanity of sorts, and regained sanity a state of deluded conformity? At least the speaker has emerged from 'cells of madness, haunts of horror and fear' (part 3, stanza 1); but is his new-found ability to use the first-person plural – 'We have proved we have hearts in a cause, we are noble still' (part 3, stanza 5) – a sign of health or a jump from frying-pan to fire? It is arguable that the poem explores those 'haunts of horror and fear' with rather more conviction than it suggests that the speaker is objectively right in his final analysis. Indeed, section 3 captures well the release from anxiety and complication that war in a cause deemed to be 'noble' often seems to offer.

For many twentieth-century poets, madness opposes to itself to sanity as protest to wrong, as in Yeats's 'Why should not old men be mad?' Experience, Yeats snarls in this poem, presents so much that is contradictory and disappointing that madness feels like a kick against misery: 'Some think it a matter of course that chance / Should starve good men and bad advance, / That if their neighbours figured plain / As though upon a lighted screen, / No single story would they find / Of an unbroken happy mind, / A finish worthy of the start. / Young men know nothing of this sort, / Observant old men know it well'.[19] These embittered reflections deploy rhymes that grow slant ('plain'/ 'screen'; 'start'/'sort'). The poem's last line ('Know why an old man should be mad') circles back to the first line ('Why should not old men be mad?') with the insistent, even maddened emphasis often found in poetic representations of madness. Yeats both assumes and resists the role of mad poet. If he is Crazy Jane in some lyrics, or if the poem just quoted was first published in *On the Boiler*, a volume in which he expounds some of his most reactionary, eugenicist ideas and which takes its title from his hearing as a boy a '"mad ship's carpenter" speaking on top of a large, rusted boiler, "denounc[ing] his neighbours"', there is an exalted terror in his work at the thought of a collective descent into chaos.[20] 'A civilisation is a struggle to keep self-control,' he writes in *A Vision*, 'and in this it is like some great tragic person, some Niobe who must display an almost superhuman will or the cry will not touch our sympathy. The loss of control over thought comes towards the end; first a sinking in upon the moral being, then the last surrender, the irrational cry, revelation – the scream of Juno's peacock'.[21] As 'revelation' suggests, terror mingles with a kind of chastened exultation at the inevitable turning of the cycles, or gyres. Civilisation facing chaos is like 'some tragic person' facing personal disaster.

Madness haunts the ruin-scored echo-chamber of T. S. Eliot's *The Waste Land*. Distinctly if distantly descended from the dramatic monologue, this is a poem in which there are many speakers, melting and fragmenting, blurring and ghosting, composing something not unlike the mind – and unconscious – of Europe. That the poem's composition was connected with a breakdown on Eliot's part is well-known. But the poem works subjective sounds into its dissonant symphony of unhappy noises. At the poem's close, after the hallucinatory visions of 'What the Thunder Said', we hear a babel of voices that emerge from and bear on the speaker's attempt to shore 'fragments' of past cultures against his 'ruins'.[22] These voices include a line from Gerard de Nerval's sonnet 'El Desdischado' and allusions to Thomas Kyd's *The Spanish Tragedy* ('Why then Ile fit you. Hieronymo's mad againe') before the poem concludes with 'Shantih shantih shantih', 'a formal ending to a Upanishad', as Eliot's note instructs us. As throughout the poem, allusion works potently; Eliot mimes a general state of cultural disintegration akin to madness.

In the process of exploring the complex workings of the allusions to Kyd, Gareth Reeves asks a crucial question about the poem's close: 'Does *The Waste Land* self-destruct into fragments at its end, or does it intimate coherences yet to be achieved?'[23] Two points are worth making here. The first concerns pronouns. The words that provide this chapter's title, quoted by Eliot, come from *The Spanish Tragedy*, where Hieronimo assures the lords at court that he can 'fit' them with a play (it turns out to be the means of carrying out his revenge); 'Why then I'll fit you' has a manifest and a latent meaning, as J. R. Mulryne's editorial gloss brings out. Mulryne paraphrases Hieronimo's words at IV. I. 70 as 'I'll provide you what you need' (the manifest meaning) or 'I'll punish you as you deserve' (the latent meaning).[24] This second, more aggressive sense suits the troubled interplay between the composite narrative consciousness of Eliot's poem and the reader, left sifting through the shored-up fragments, the narrator's 'hypocrite lecteur', double and friend. The 'I' of 'Why then Ile fit you' in *The Waste Land* comes across as not wholly distinguishable from an authorial self. A doubling occurs that allows a very impersonal poem to speak with startlingly direct assertiveness. We are 'fitted ' by the poem's consciousness, which tricks out for our benefit the dishevelled echoes of lost cultural grandeur. In so fitting us, the poem virtually has a fit – and immediately breaks off into madness ('Hieronymo's mad againe') and is only seconds away from the silence that Kyd's Hieronimo will himself choose (he bites out his tongue) and that serves as madness's authenticating sign.

The second point to be made about the allusions to Kyd concerns the line's function in its context. Lyndall Gordon makes a shrewd observation about the revision of this passage. 'In the first draft', she argues, 'the allusion to Hieronimo's madness comes after the allusion to Arnaut Daniel and is therefore one of the fragments the wanderer shores against his ruins. In the next draft Eliot ... moves Hieronimo further on. In its transposed position the line has a different effect. It suggests not recovery but the babblings of encroaching madness'.[25] Admittedly, 'Shantih shantih shantih' offers an ambiguously transcendental alternative, but Gordon's point holds true of the poem. Words that remind us of Hieronimo's orchestrating competence remind us more of the destructive, vengeful motives that lie behind that competence. In its turn, Eliot's poem takes revenge on a culture and readership prepared to sanitise itself with dreams of order. The conclusion of *The Waste Land* hovers between break-down and break-through.

The Waste Land has a modernist last-stand quality about it, as though Eliot were pronouncing on the end of civilisation as he or we had known it. In later poems, psychic disintegration flirts with an unmediated capacity to shock. This chapter will conclude with analyses of poems by three major American poets, all associated with mental disorder, psychiatry, bipolar mental states especially manic depression, and 'so-called' confessional poetry: Robert Lowell, John Berryman, and Sylvia Plath. Lowell's poems about mental breakdown in *Life Studies* represent a major poetic innovation less because they deal with hitherto taboo subject-matter without recourse to persona or drama than because they manage to make personal anguish into art. In 'Skunk Hour', the confessional heart of the poem is the line 'My mind's not right', but it is in the travelling towards and away from this declaration that the poem's distinction resides.[26] Lowell contrives a wry, depressed but observant tone as he offers thumbnail sketches of various inhabitants from the place he is talking about (the Castine, a New England summer resort): all of them seem to inhabit an 'air / of lost connections', to quote from 'Memories of West Street and Lepke', another poem in *Life Studies*. In 'Skunk Hour', this sense of lost connections informs the slumped impact of true and slant rhymes: the hermit-heiress buys up 'all / the eyesores facing her shore/ and lets them fall'; a 'fairy' (homosexual) decorator 'brightens his shop for fall', but 'there is no money in his work, / he'd rather marry'.

The social notations catch a New England world in decline, but, subtly, Lowell suggests that their disillusion reflects his own depression, as he swings round to himself, via a grimly funny allusion to John of the Cross: 'One dark night, / my Tudor Ford climbed the hill's skull, / I watched for love-cars'. The poet as excluded voyeur sees the landscape as a giant skull, linking sex with death (the love cars lay 'where the graveyard shelves on the town'). The effect is of a man who dawningly recognises that his 'mind's not right', watching himself watching others with enough acuteness to suggest that the wrongness of his mind results in a disturbing rightness of perception. It is another poem 'trembling on the brink of madness' – or not so much 'trembling' as laconically poised. 'I hear / my ill-spirit sob in each blood cell' is Lowell's response to hearing 'Love, O careless Love' on a car radio: This 'ill spirit' makes personal the earlier 'The season's ill'; it sparks off a descent into Satanic or Faustian echo: 'I myself am hell'. And yet, at this point of uneasy flirtation with high tragedy, the poem breaks away from personal intensities to notice 'skunks' that 'march on their soles up Main Street'. Those 'soles' are jokily physical (there is no concern with spiritual 'souls' in skunkland), and the skunks offer the poet something like an emblem of animal will to survive, a sub- or non-human courage that bears ambiguously on the poet's state of mind. For instance, you could see the final image of the mother skunk that 'jabs her wedge head in a cup / of sour cream, drops her ostrich tail, / and will not scare' as strangely heartening; or as showing that the poet, by contrast, does 'scare' (himself and others). The poet is left, at the end, still watching. There is a weightless, topsy-turvy feel. Possibly the focus on the skunks is ostrich-like, a way of hiding from mental suffering, and yet the man is grateful to be shunted from centre-stage by the animals. The poem amuses itself by allowing the earlier mother of a bishop (the hermit-heiress) to be usurped by the mother of the skunks. Minimal consolations – the mother skunk's courage – float as possibilities; otherness may just help as well as confirm the self's isolation.

Otherness as a refuge is less apparent in Sylvia Plath. According to Philip Larkin, 'Mad poets do not write about madness: they write about religion, sofas, the French Revolution, nature, their cat Jeoffry. Plath did: it was her subject ... together they played an increasingly reckless game of tag'.[27] Perhaps; but there is much validity in views of Plath which stress the poetry's cunning self-awareness. Jacqueline Rose argues, for example, that Plath's most seemingly distraught poem – 'Daddy' – is 'a poem about its own conditions of linguistic and phantasmic production'.[28] She has in mind the way Plath enacts the moving towards identification with a persecuted Jew, as if showing us the complex working-out of cultural fantasy; 'I think I may well be a Jew', 'I may be a bit of a Jew'.[29] Anthony Easthope opposes this view and finds 'Daddy' to be a 'humanist poem, and a pretty old-fashioned one', which offers 'a dramatisation of the unified self'.[30] My position is somewhere in between: Rose may too quickly remove Plath from personal involvement, Easthope too quickly deny her anything else. In 'Daddy', Plath supplies a searing example of the split between tortured experience and formal control. The poem almost sends up the drive towards insistent rhyme in many poems concerning 'madness' as it repeats over and over, in sickening nursery-rhyme-like chant, its 'oo' sound. Moreover, the terrifying discovery of the self's isolation found in Clare's 'I Am' or in Tennyson's *Maud* reappears here as virtual mockery; the very pronoun 'I' flaunts both its unignorable insistence and its unsayability when translated into German: 'I never could talk to you. / The tongue stuck in my jaw. / It stuck in a barb wire snare. / Ich, ich, ich, ich, / I could hardly speak'. If the poem exultantly overcomes suppression of speech, as it gets through to the father-figure, the last line, 'Daddy, daddy, you bastard, I'm through', contains the flattened suggestion that the self is done with, finished, defeated. Plath seems at once identical with and aloof from her speaker, and that dance of intimacy and distance between poet and speaker is as powerful a relationship as the relationship between speaker and father which is the poem's explicit subject. Yet, to read it solely as a poem watching itself is to deny the source of its power; the feeling that it dramatises a clairvoyant, lost self spinning round a sense of being damaged, longing in equal measure for revenge on and connection with the father.

There is comedy of a bleakly mirthless kind in Plath. There is comedy, too, in the poetry of John Berryman, whose *Dream Songs* are a poetry impossible to imagine before Freud. In these poems Berryman finds a language for the psyche, frequently veering between sonorous diction and slang, achieving, as Lowell and Plath do, a way of talking about the world even as he explores the depths of the self. One of Berryman's tricks is to escape the confessional by creating a fictional persona called 'Henry' who is sometimes addressed, in vaudeville-style language, by an unnamed interlocutor. And yet it is a relatively straightforward elegy with which I wish to finish this chapter, Berryman's elegy for a poet, the gifted, doomed Delmore Schwartz. In Lowell's 'To Delmore Schwartz', Schwartz is ventriloquised as wittily rewriting Wordsworth's 'Resolution and Independence': 'We poets in our youth begin in sadness; / thereof in the end comes despondency and madness; / Stalin has had two cerebral haemorrages!'. Seizing on Stalin – the very type of anti-poetry – as the typical poet is ruefully witty about poetry's own forms of despotic control. Berryman wrote a series of poems about Schwartz after his death, celebrating his youthful genius and lamenting his wasted talents, including the following, 'Dream Song 147':

> Henry's mind grew blacker the more he thought.
> He looked onto the world like the act of an aged whore.
> Delmore, Delmore.
> He flung to pieces and they hit the floor.
> Nothing was true but what Marcus Aurelius taught,
> 'All that is foul smell & blood in a bag.'
>
> He lookt on the world like the leavings of a hag,
> Almost his love died from him, any more.
> His mother & William
> were vivid in the same mail Delmore died.
> The world is lunatic. This is the last ride.
> Delmore, Delmore.
>
> High in the summer branches the poet sang.
> His throat ached, and he could sing no more.
> All ears closed
> across the heights where Delmore & Gertrude sprang
> so long ago, in the goodness of which it was composed.
> Delmore, Delmore![31]

The poem pivots on the dead poet's first name, repeated like a refrain, the last time with a speech-defeated exclamation mark. 'Delmore' dominates the rhyming. This 'despotic' rhyming (to borrow Coleridge's adjective) shows the poet coming back to the one thought. Pulling against this centripetal movement is a scattering, best caught in the line: 'He flung to pieces and they hit the floor', where Henry – as throughout the poem – breaks up (as well as down). This two-way process foments the poem's whirling between past ('He lookt on the world ...') and present ('The world is lunatic'). It shows itself in the clash between grief at the loss of male friendship and the battily down-at-heel, Lear-like raging against the world as a sexually promiscuous woman (though Henry's own looking could be so described as a result of the slippery syntax). It can be heard, too, in the movement between the consolations of pent-up anger and the sense that such anger will have its day, a movement audible in the words, 'This is the last ride', which contrive to sound final and to concede that they are not. Moreover, it is a process at work in the pull between Henry's distress and the assertion that it is 'the world' which is 'lunatic'. The world's lunacy consists in the crazy contingency of events; Henry gets 'vivid' letters from 'Mother & William' in the same postal delivery as the news of his friend's death. Henry recognises such lunacy, too, in the cruel depredations of time that can turn the long-ago 'goodness' into 'foul smell & blood in a bag', and that bring even grief to an end: 'His throat ached and he could sing no more'. His poetic 'ears' begin to be 'closed' to memories, even though it is with memories that the poem 'closes'.

Shaping all these tensions and pulls is a voice that relies on, even as it redefines, poetic form. In Berryman's elegy, as often in poems about, or sensing the proximity of, madness, the use of poetic form asserts a residual belief in order. It is not an order, however, that is antagonistic to disorder. Formal order for Berryman, as for the other poets discussed in this chapter, suffers with mental disorder, offering a sympathy from which emerges, to use a word significantly placed near this poem's end, something 'composed'.

Notes

1 Quoted from *Samuel Taylor Coleridge*, Oxford Authors, ed. H. J. Jackson (Oxford, 1985), p. 602.
2 Coleridge, pp. 408, 409.
3 See Peter Barham, *Closing the Asylum: The Mental Patient in Modern Society*, 2nd edn (Harmondsworth, 1997), p. 171.
4 Quoted from *Byron*, Oxford Authors, ed. Jerome J. McGann (Oxford, 1986).
5 Quoted from Elizabeth Jennings, *Collected Poems 1953–1985* (Manchester, 1986).
6 Quoted from *John Clare*, Oxford Authors, ed. Eric Robinson and David Powell (Oxford, 1984).
7 Jacques Derrida, *Writing and Difference*, trans. with intro. Alan Bass (London, 1978), p. 36.
8 Poem and Preface are quoted from *Percy Bysshe Shelley: The Major Works*, ed. Zachary Leader and Michael O'Neill (Oxford, 2003). For a discussion of madness and Romanticism, see Frederick Burwick, *Poetic Madness and the Romantic Imagination* (University Park, PA, 1996).
9 Roy Porter, *The Greatest Benefit to Mankind: A Medical History of Humanity from Antiquity to the Present* (London, 1997), p. 495.

10 'The Dramatic Monologue in the Victorian Period', *Proceedings of the British Academy 1924–1925*, p. 276.

11 Quoted from *Robert Browning's Poetry: Authoritative Texts, Criticism*, ed. James F. Loucks (New York, 1979).

12 Loucks, pp. 525, 526.

13 Loucks, p. 526.

14 See *The Poems of Browning, volume 1: 1826–1840*, ed. John Woolford and Daniel Karlin (London, 1991), p. 331.

15 Woolford and Karlin, p. 329.

16 Quoted, as is the text of the poem, from *The Poems of Tennyson*, ed. Christopher Ricks (London, 1969), p. 1039.

17 Christopher Ricks, *Tennyson* (1972, London, 1978 rpt. with alterations), p. 259.

18 Ricks, p. 259.

19 Quoted from *Yeats's Poems*, ed. A. Norman Jeffares, with an appendix by Warwick Gould (London, 1989).

20 Quoted from *W. B. Yeats: The Poems*, ed. Daniel Albright (London, 1994), p. 804.

21 Quoted from W. B. Yeats, *A Vision* (1937; London, 1962), p. 268.

22 All quotations from the text of and Eliot's notes to *The Waste Land* are taken from the text of the first 1922 edition printed in *The Waste Land: A Facsimile and Transcript of the Original Drafts Including the Annotations of Ezra Pound*, ed. Valerie Eliot (London, 1971).

23 Gareth Reeves, *T. S. Eliot's 'The Waste Land'* (Hemel Hempstead, 1994), p. 99.

24 Thomas Kyd, *The Spanish Tragedy*, ed. J. R. Mulryne (London, 1970), p. 105.

25 Lyndall Gordon, *Eliot's Early Years* (Oxford, 1977), p. 115.

26 Quoted, as are all poems by Lowell, from his *Life Studies*, 2nd edn (London, 1968).

27 Philip Larkin, 'Horror Poet', in his *Required Writing: Miscellaneous Pieces 1955–1982* (London, 1983), p. 281.

28 Jacqueline Rose, *The Haunting of Sylvia Plath* (London, 1991), p. 230.

29 Quoted from Sylvia Plath, *Ariel* (1965, London, 1968).

30 Antony Easthope, 'Reading the Poetry of Sylvia Plath', *English* 43 (Autumn 1994), pp. 223–35; quoted from *The Poetry of Sylvia Plath: A Reader's Guide to Essential Criticism*, ed. Claire Brennan (Cambridge, 2000), p. 149.

31 Quoted from John Berryman, *The Dream Songs* (London, 1990).

9

Madness, Medicine and Creativity in Thomas Mann's *The Magic Mountain*

Martyn Evans

Introduction

To attempt, in just a few pages, to explore ideas of madness and creativity in the context of so celebrated yet so daunting an epic as Thomas Mann's *The Magic Mountain* seems like a perilous quest – a quest with its own undertones of faint madness (in conception) and an abundant need for creativity (in execution). This arises not least because our considerations must be developed on the basis of a synopsis of the novel; such a synopsis has somehow to avoid seeming either indecently sketchy to those readers who know the work well, or intimidatingly congested to those readers who do not.

I will start by putting the novel in context and giving a flavour of it at first encounter. Then I shall set out what I think are the 'big questions' with which the book is ostensibly concerned. As they stand, these 'big questions' could easily claim our attention on their own terms. Yet they do not straightforwardly fit the central themes of this volume – or, at least, not without a little work. I will therefore harness these questions to three *conjectures* that are more transparently relevant to this volume's concerns. I think these conjectures are plausibly discerned in the book, and that they may plausibly appeal to the professional palates of doctors, psychiatrists, historians and philosophers, as well as to the palates of those who love literature for its own sake. In each case, I shall try to show in a little more detail how these conjectures can be pursued in the book, and in its 'big questions'.

Context and content

The Magic Mountain has been described as 'the epic of disease'.[1] It is certainly of epic length – more than seven hundred pages in a standard English translation[2] – and it charts a seven-year voyage, of an unusual kind: a stationary voyage of self-discovery, in a suitably remote and in many ways exotic location, with a company of the oddest shipmates, surrounded immediately by the physical and moral dangers of a rather luxurious form of chronic disease; just over the horizon, the continent of Europe is preparing to tear itself apart in war.

Clearly an epic, then, given its scale and the imposing backdrop; an epic moreover *of disease* in that the voyage of self-discovery (about which we shall say more) is a voyage into, and amidst, disease – disease as a physical, psychological, moral and cultural phenomenon. Mann described himself as a chronicler and analyst of decadence,[3] and one of his interests here is in disease as an expression of decadence, a vehicle, an arena for decadence. Of course, not just any disease will do – it has to be one which is culturally and symbolically powerful, and whose course lasts long enough to allow its victims to be interesting. If Mann were writing today, then the chosen disease might have been cancer, or parkinsonism, or AIDS. In the early years of the twentieth century it happened to be tuberculosis – the 'consumption' which so fixated the fear and fascination of the Victorians and their immediate successors.[4]

The sheer physical size of the book suggests it is in some sense 'important', yet to engage it casually is, initially, to be daunted by its sheer bulk, its quaint, stilted style, its somewhat remote characters, its endless philosophising, and its unbelievably slow action – the protracted meals, inconsequential walks and cerebral talk, occasionally spiced up by suppressed eroticism. I recall my own first reactions to the book. After the promising opening pages, set on a narrow-gauge steam railway (a winning *entrée* to an adventure yarn, perhaps), I soon found myself mired in baffling flashbacks, then stuck in the time-warp of a hotel where it seemed absolutely nothing happened whatsoever. After a hundred pages of this, I was still trudging through chapters with titles like 'Table talk' or 'Soup everlasting'. Then things seemed to pick up quite sharply at around a third of the way through the book, in a chapter intriguingly called 'Sudden enlightenment'. And then from there I was intermittently electrified – brought face to face with some of the biggest ideas anyone could possibly think about. The book *becomes* a sort of magic mountain – massive, enveloping, beguiling, hypnotic, exhausting to negotiate but somehow also transforming. As happens to its principal character in one of the pivotal set-piece scenes, the book leads you to a kind of summit, then dumps you back into the daily round of ordinary living with sometimes only a vague sense of what it was you thought you'd grasped so clearly in the previous evening's reading.

The novel's 'big questions'

What is the book about? What is it meant to tell us? Why does it take the form it takes? And why should we pay attention to it? On the largest scale it is tempting to say the book is about the meaning of life: that is to say, the very largest questions about our experience, our knowledge, our embodied nature, our culture. On the smallest scale it is about a few years in the self-absorbed growing up of a bored young man, his first adventures in love, and his attempts to come to terms with the people who want to influence his thoughts. Midway between these, it is about the perilous charms of indulgent Romanticist thought, the ambiguity of beauty and decay, and the balance between the biological and the biographical in disease causation, all mingled for good measure with the influence of a cultural and intellectual fascination with psychoanalysis. On yet a different level the book is about literature itself, an essay in the stretching of a particular literary convention (the *Bildungsroman* or novel of educational and spiritual development, an important theme in German Romantic literature).[5] And on this same level it is also about exploring the effects of using very large, very extended metaphors. In more concrete terms, the whole course of the book concerns the enmity and struggle between life and death. Superficially healthy people of all ages come to the Mountain retreat in order to fall sick and, very often, to die – trying to get as much fun (usually trivial) as possible while they are doing it. They dwell on this grim truth about themselves, yet they also hide from it. The book implicitly condemns them as blind, spoilt children – just very occasionally it invites our pity for them, as the frightened victims of irresistible disease.

But at specific points in the book we also start to explore the practical realities and the *philosophical* dimensions of this larger concern with the meaning of life and death. For instance in that attention-grabbing chapter I mentioned earlier, the one called 'Sudden illumination', we see the book's fragile hero, Hans Castorp, encountering for the first time his own bodiliness, and thus his mortality, when he sees a vision of his own skeleton, the bones of his hand in the primitive fluoroscope machine. This is the scene, electrifying even in translation:

A few minutes later [Hans Castorp] himself stood in the pillory, in the midst of the electrical storm, while Joachim, his body closed up again, put on his clothes. Again the Hofrat peered into the milky glass, this time into Hans Castorp's own inside; and from his half-utterances, his broken phrases and bursts of scolding, the young man gathered that what he saw corresponded to his expectations. He was so kind as to permit the patient, at his request, to look at his own hand through the screen. And Hans Castorp saw, precisely what he must have expected, but what it is hardly permitted man to see, and what he thought it would never be vouchsafed him to see: he looked into his own grave. The process of decay was forestalled by the powers of the light-ray, the flesh in which he walked disintegrated, annihilated, dissolved in vacant mist, and there within it was the finely turned skeleton of his own hand, the seal ring he had inherited from his grandfather hanging loose and black on the joint of his ring-finger – a hard, material object with which man adorns the body that is fated to melt away beneath it, when it passes on to another flesh that can wear it for yet a little while. ...[With] penetrating, prophetic eyes, he gazed at this familiar part of his own body, and for the first time in his life he understood that he would die.[6]

From this point on, Hans starts to dwell on how health, flourishing, love, sickness and death somehow belong together. He starts to get to grips with the idea that death has both an 'indecent and a sacred aspect', an idea which leads him into mortal peril – physically as well as spiritually or morally. And his moral grip on the different claims of life and death is tested to the full, late on in the book, by the apparently occult 'reappearance' of his dead cousin Joachim at a séance. Indeed over the course of the book Hans Castorp looks metaphorically into his own grave through the fluoroscope machine, physically into Joachim's grave at his cousin's funeral, and (supernaturally? It is never made quite clear) *beyond* Joachim's grave at a séance.

Perhaps not surprisingly, all of this provides Thomas Mann with ample material for a re-working of the Faust legend, exploring a man's craving for secret, forbidden knowledge of life and death, and his willingness to risk almost anything in order to get it (and not only here in *The Magic Mountain* but also in the later, and morally less ambiguous *Doctor Faustus* where the diabolic pact concerns musical rather than philosophical insight).[7]

The dangers of such a bargain for Hans Castorp are moral and intellectual as well as physical. Not only does he court bodily death out in the open, when illicitly skiing on the mountain's uncharted upper slopes in search of self-knowledge: in his indoor adventures into moral peril, there is more than a hint of necrophilia tainting his adventurous erotic fixation for fellow-patient Clavdia Chauchat, the beautiful Russian émigré whom he desires to *know* (as he puts it) 'under the skin'. His superficially scientific interest in human anatomy is erotically projected onto Clavdia. In the important chapters describing his thirst for book-knowledge, he builds up in his mind a 'dissection' of the material universe and of humanity's place within it, and this leads to his assembling in his feverish imagination a sort of animated corpse who takes on Clavdia's form and features.

These passages, crafted by Mann with disturbing conviction, raise a very large question. To announce it, let me ask a small question: Why a woman like the feline Clavdia? To which the answer is, I believe, that erotic love (to give Hans Castorp's dubious fixation the benefit of the doubt) vividly raises the philosophical conundrum of whether the connection between personality and embodiment is a necessary or an accidental one. The philosopher Hans Jonas once memorably averred that when he fell in love with his wife, it was not with her brain.[8] Whilst such a remark sounds rather like the strategic conversational weapon of last resort, Jonas was not being offensively sexist; as the context makes clear, he meant simply that humans come in complete physical and mental packages, from which the personality cannot be as it were 'hived off'; the ghost cannot be isolated, still less exorcised, from the machine. There are few bigger questions from the standpoint of philosophy, psychiatry or somatic medicine than what is conventionally called the 'mind-body problem'. In medical terms, at stake are the causal relations amongst psychological and patho-physiological states, an intensely topical concern for us in the Genome Age. Mann overtly pursues the idea that our bodily health is inseparable from what we might call our 'narrative selves', and that there is more to us than biology alone – with a (for him) contemporary twist in the phenomenal advance of Freudian psychoanalysis, explored through the Svengali-like figure of the rather dirty-minded analyst, Dr. Krokowski. Perhaps, like Karl Popper more recently, Mann felt that psychoanalysis was doubly bogus for presenting what was really a belief system as if it were a way of doing science.[9] At any rate, he gives it a good kicking, via the unfortunate backside of the miserable Krokowski.

There are many specific invitations in the book to think about the mind-body relation and the influence of the mind on bodily health and disease. For one, Hans Castorp several times enters an odd mental state, usually a fevered imagining, that employs some connection between certain kinds of vision and bodily effects (a nosebleed, a fever, the 'rush' of nicotine, and so forth). For another, the sanatorium's medical director (the *Hofrat*) considers that his patients' health is sometimes governed by their wishes and intentions. He openly accuses Hans Castorp's cousin Joachim of a death wish, springing from his austere sense of military honour.

For a third, Hans Castorp himself regards a certain decorous degree of physical ill-health as an integral part of the aesthetic detachment needed for true intellectual enlightenment (a faintly mad conviction, we might think, in the service of his quest for creativity. In this he foreshadows the acceptance, by the central character in *Doctor Faustus*, the composer Leverkuhn, of mortification via the wilful contracting of disease as part of the price of creativity).[10] There is method in Hans Castorp's madness, of course – illness *is* a meal-ticket at the sanatorium. Moreover, his illness is so gentle, so conjectural, as to be a very easily-tolerated 'mortification of the flesh', and one obtained without having to summon the moral courage to inflict it himself; instead of to a scourge, he submits merely to a regime of being pampered.

Other invitations to reflect on the mind-body problem permeate the entire novel. We are offered, throughout one of the novel's sub-plots, a recurrent theme of the idea of sickness in cultural and intellectual states of affairs. These are largely centred around the sinister Jesuitical figure of Naphta: the sort of blind authoritarian society he wants is presented, by

Mann's (seemingly) approved spokesmen, as a form of cultural illness. And for all the novel's moral ambiguity, Hans Castorp's 'Faustian' curiosity is more-or-less openly branded an intellectual disease by the time we reach the closing pages. This is, of course, a nightmarishly-quick review of some of the 'big questions' with which the novel is concerned. If we summed them up under 'the meaning of life', we would be being glib – but not wildly inaccurate. Hans Castorp wants to discover precisely the meaning of life, just as we all do. It is Mann's particularly Puckish twist on all of this that he should envelop, indeed strap up, such questions within the corsets of the conventional German Romantic literary form of a *Bildungsroman*. Thus we engage Castorp's spiritual journey of adventure and discovery, beginning with his retreat away from the bourgeois anonymity of Hamburg, down in the 'Flatlands', up to the rarefied Mountain. Intellectually, morally and spiritually we are invited to watch his fall and, ultimately, his apparent resurrection. Initially he is naïve, wishing to absorb all possible influences prior to challenging them as his confidence grows. Later he will reject the simplistic association between love and death as false; reject the 'attractions' of disease; reject the 'questionable' occult; reject the Mountain itself, finally; and wake up to obey a different calling – the call to arms in the First World War.

Much of this story of awakening and enlightenment proceeds via the eminently suitable grand-metaphor of *vision*, exploited to huge effect in both physical and metaphorical presentations including illusion and deception (including *self*-deception, of course). A *chain* of visual illusion haunts Hans Castorp, unifying experiences as diverse as those of his grandfather's grave, the apparition of a school friend, a mystical near-death experience in a snowstorm, and reflections of his dead cousin from beyond the grave, most grossly at a séance. These are counterpoised, intriguingly, by literal or physical visions including those of the X-ray machine and its products, and the painted and the X-ray 'portraits' of his *amour*. I think every comic genre from the silent film right through to the Simpsons would gladly make room for the deliciously Goonish folly of an infatuated young man carrying round a *really* naughty picture of his heart's desire in his inside jacket pocket; how much more nude can you get than an X-ray picture – yet how much less erotic? Throughout, we are teased with the idea that penetrative vision entails penetrative understanding, even penetrative possession: yet how readily we might now reflect that modern biomedicine thrives on the supposition that the real somehow *underlies* the superficial, at the same time devoting its technological resources to making the unseen become seen, to making hidden structures visible![11]

This is an example of how Thomas Mann *inverts* so many of his readers' expectations that he could be said to invert the way his *Bildungsroman* and its grand metaphors secure their effect. The shocking twist of course is that the Mountain *does* offer an awakening that Castorp could not obtain in his conventional life – and *disease* itself partly offers this awakening (this 'resurrection'). Mann's artful rejection of the Romantic convention that 'disease is interesting' consists as much in showing what Hans Castorp learns through rejecting it, as it does in having affectionate fun at Hans Castorp's expense whilst he is still in its insane grip.

And finally, just for good measure, consider the parallels between the snowbound Mountain sanatorium and a sinking lifeboat – and then consider the stock characters with which the lifeboat is supplied, the huffing, puffing, purple-cheeked authority figure, the clean-cut officer cadet, the idealistic youth, the *femme fatale*, the various buffoons, the sinister manipulator and so on: all the ingredients of the slightly later cinematic cliché, the 'disaster-movie'. What distinguishes Mann's novel from cheap cinema is of course not simply the former's high-art context, its emotional subtlety, the philosophical gravity of its ideas and action or the ingenuity and sophistication of its narrative structure, but also the grandeur of the language employed to convey all of these. Even in translation, the form of ideas in literature dominates their content – the words are powerful beyond their literal meaning.

> ... And to the pulsation of the floor, and the snapping and cracking of the forces at play, Hans Castorp peered through the lighted window, peered into Joachim Ziemssen's empty skeleton. The breastbone and spine fell together in a single dark column. The frontal structure of the ribs was cut across by the paler structure of the back. Above, the collarbones branched off on both sides, and the framework of the shoulder, with the joint and the beginning of Joachim's arm, showed sharp and bare through the soft envelope of flesh...
>
> ...But Hans Castorp's attention was taken up by something like a bag, a strange, animal shape, darkly visible behind the middle column, or more on the right side of it – the spectator's right. It expanded and contracted regularly, a little after the fashion of a swimming jelly-fish.
>
> 'Look at his heart,' and the Hofrat lifted his huge hand again from his thigh and pointed with his forefinger at the pulsating shadow. Good God, it was the heart, it was Joachim's honour-loving heart that Hans Castorp saw![12]

I have tried to draw attention to some of the 'big questions' with which *The Magic Mountain* is occupied – to summarise, they include the mind-body relation; the mixture of the biological and the biographical in our health and our sickness; the enmity between life and death and the decadence of being drawn to death; the perils of the Faustian bargain; and so forth. But as I mentioned at the outset, interesting though these overt themes are, they do not all equally claim our attention within the terms of reference of the present volume.

So let me proceed now to suggest three 'conjectures' which I think Mann implicitly offers us in *The Magic Mountain*, and which *do* claim the attention of anyone interested in madness, the mind, creativity and medicine.

Three conjectures

My conjectures are as follows, in simple terms:

The first is that the relation between mind and body is illuminated, perhaps especially brightly, by *pathology* or *disease*. In particular, bodily pathology reflects and expresses pathology arising in other terms – personal, psychological, social, or cultural.

The second, arising from the first, is that madness can be a manifestation of cultural decadence, identified as such in moral, aesthetic and intellectual terms. Such decadence is, in *The Magic Mountain*, distinguished by contrast with reason, and it is reversible (or 'curable') by means of a partly moral struggle.

The third conjecture is that *creativity itself* is a mystery, a kind of darkness, in cosmic terms something morally ambiguous, for which we (or Hans?) must continually struggle in moral as well as physical and intellectual terms (a theme to which Mann returns in the later *Doctor Faustus*).

There is a fourth as well, perhaps, which I have not space to develop here. But since it concerns medicine, let me at least mention it before passing on: it is that in Mann's terms, medicine is a *technologising* of processes which it *assumes* to be physical but which are in reality at least partly moral, intellectual or aesthetic. Interestingly, that fourth conjecture is perhaps far less radical now than when the novel was written. Even so, it would command our attention were there space here to consider it; but since we have not, I shall leave it here, and confine myself to the first three.

The mind-body question

First, then, the mind-body question. For Thomas Mann as the 'poet and chronicler of decadence', decadence has a natural physical outlet in bodily disease, and a tailor-made literary and metaphorical outlet in a culturally-interesting specific disease such as tuberculosis. Of course, disease has been used as an extended metaphor for decadence before – in Shakespeare's *Hamlet*, for instance, where we first encounter 'something rotten in the state of Denmark'. The difference is that in *The Magic Mountain* we sense that Mann is more interested in using decadence to explore disease, rather than the other way around.

Beyond this, disease is the prism through which Mann considers the intertwining of mind and body in the human condition. The personality, if you like, expresses the limitations of the body – including those limitations placed upon it 'externally' by contracting a disease like tuberculosis.

Disease and decadence indicate or disclose one another. In current parlance, each is part of the other's 'evidence base'.

We have already noticed some of the hints Mann drops in this regard – cousin Joachim's 'death-wish', Hans Castorp's desire to be admitted to the ranks of the decorously-sick. But there are other, more extended and developed variations on the mind-body tune, of which two are worth our noticing now. Both concern things which (I think) Mann invites us to disapprove, namely the attempted *reduction* of mind to body, and the attempted *suppression* of mind *by* body.[13] Though related, these are actually two quite distinct ideas. The reduction of mind to body implies that mind disappears as a distinct phenomenon; it is dissolved, leaving no residue. By contrast, its suppression implies that it retains a subordinate, but nonetheless still real, position in the moral universe. In order to recruit our disapproval in each case, Mann places these two assaults on mind in the hands of multiple proponents who are variously comical or sinister.

The sanatorium's medical director, Herr Hofrat Behrens, is deliciously-drawn, a mixture of the urbane and the prickly, the artful and the bluff, the decent man of science and the lascivious old lecher. He provides us – and Hans Castorp – with endless opportunity for speculation concerning his relations with the alluring Mme. Clavdia Chauchat, be they in the consulting room, the X-ray suite or his private portrait-painting studio. At one point he and Hans discuss his amateurish portrait of Clavdia, in which both men have an interest that is decidedly ambiguous. For Behrens, the portrait succeeds in as much as it captures her womanliness in the constitutive structure of her skin and its fatty 'upholstering'. For Hans Castorp, the portrait succeeds in being a simple *token* of her presence in the room with them. Both agree (or at least, pretend to agree) that a painting can succeed in performing a kind of anatomy, in which the personal magnetism of their feline *femme fatale* can be reduced to a kind of physiological analysis.[14]

This leads them on to a short discussion of psycho-somatic phenomena including goose-pimples, and the variety of means by which they can be produced. The terms of their discussion happen to interest me personally because I am fond of beginning my own introductory lectures on the mind-body question by *describing* – though *not* demonstrating – the scraping of fingernails down a blackboard and inviting the students to give as full an account as they can of their response to my descriptions. The idea, of course, is to show how even such unambiguously mental events as verbal descriptions can have an amusingly causal role in physio-mechanical processes. (I am pleased to report that the results induced among one's audience are normally gratifying to the malevolent lecturer.)

Hofrat Behrens would roundly approve. Just prior to one of the novel's best comic moments, he invites Hans Castorp to imagine having a bucketful of minnows in cold water poured over him, like the young man in the fable who wanted to know what it was like to shiver. This isn't quite high-flown enough for Hans, who responds that *he* gets goose-pimples from church music, and from taking communion. 'Oh,' responds Behrens, in what must set new standards for deflationary comparison, 'tickling's tickling. The body doesn't give a hang for the content of the stimulus. It may be minnows, it may be the Holy Ghost, the sebaceous glands are erected just the same.'[15]

Another largely comic character is the retired Dutch colonial, Pieter Peeperkorn, who is the only one of the novel's would-be demagogues to succeed in regularly 'wowing' an audience – despite also being the only one of the three to be incapable of finishing a coherent sentence even when sober, which is not often. Peeperkorn is larger-than-life in most senses, and indeed he is – or stands for – a kind of animalism, a sort of vital-principle-on-legs, for whom gigantic fleshly appetites are the index of being truly alive.

Peeperkorn is reductionism writ large – if you will forgive that slightly paradoxical-sounding phrase. His moral force is generated in his sheer animalism: moral power just *is* physical power, merging with nature's grandeur. And curiously enough, the scrawny and ascetic young Hans Castorp feels the force of it. The young idealist – who thinks that the mind ought to emerge hurriedly from the physical and then flee away from it as far and as fast as possible – actually falls under Peeperkorn's physicalist spell.

The darker side of all this is that where the mind cannot be *reduced* to the body, it may at any rate be *suppressed* by it. Pieter Peeperkorn – who is in the business of assertion rather than explanation – can accept nothing beyond the animal powers of physicalism. When he discovers that he is sexually impotent, he concludes that he deserves to die – and die he does, by his own hand, an act for which he has clearly made careful and elaborate preparations, with exactly this circumstance in mind. No experiential longings shall be allowed to survive the demise of the means to assuage them. The view that impotence deserves death is an extreme one, particularly unusual amongst consumptive septuagenarians. In the parlance, Peeperkorn has a lot of 'attitude', but some slightly comic limitations to his imagination.

Unfortunately, the cultural equivalent of this suppression of mind by body is presented through the political brutality of the views of the book's oddest and darkest character, the Jesuitical ex-priest, Naphta. He is the constant foil to the liberal views of the social reformer, Signor Settembrini, and their interminable disputes end tragically in a pointless duel of honour, when Naphta blows out his own brains. It is a result not without its satisfactions, one feels by that stage of the book, where reason, democracy, liberty, literacy and reform have all been denigrated by Naphta in favour of conformism, the authority of church and state, the enforcement of that authority by torture and execution, and a general espousal of political and spiritual terrorism. For Naphta, individual thought is to be smashed into conformity, and radicalism suppressed by physical pain and terror: in the interests of its purification, the human spirit is to be devoured by the state, just as for Peeperkorn the human imagination is to be assimilated into bodily urges and appetites.

Any sophisticated novelist knows how to keep us, as readers, suspended while we discover his sympathies as well as our own. Mann, a Nobel laureate, is more sophisticated than most. But the suspense is, I think, resolved: the reduction and suppression of the mind *is* presented to us finally as madness, be it the folly of the buffoon or the fantasies of the psychopath.

Madness

And this takes us, then, directly into the second of my conjectures, concerning madness as such, namely that madness is largely an expression of moral and cultural decadence – and that recovery from madness is to be attained partly in moral terms. Of course, there's something basically mad about the entire situation in *The Magic Mountain*. Up on the mountain, a group of Europe's idle rich are engaged in drawing out for as long as possible the collective denial of how physically sick they are, whilst operating a social hierarchy based on precisely that sickness they deny. Too ill to ski, they dress up in skiing costume nonetheless. They would have dressed up as shepherdesses – if only sheep were more glamorous. They want to cheat Death of his prey, yet they whet his appetite by holding séances. Institutionalised medicine provides them with the justificatory rhetoric of their illness – yet also of their self-indulgence. Indeed medicine supplies the environment for that indulgence, the entertainments necessary to divert the patients, the rituals for their treatment and the priestly authority for managing their deaths discreetly and out of sight. Meanwhile, everyone else in Europe is preparing for the most public form of mutual slaughter in the First World War. As insane situations go, it is considerable.

And in the central figure of Hans Castorp we find a perfectly intelligent and decent young man whose first response to this situation is not to flee from it in disbelief, but – incredibly – to embrace it, as the invitation to a Faustian bargain concerning insights into the relative attractions of life and death. When he finally comes to his senses, *he* asserts sweet reason by quitting the Mountain in favour of the battlefield – probably to be blown to bits.

The main vehicle for Castorp's moral fall and resurrection is *vision* – both figurative and literal. As we have already noted, visual images are specifically tied to pathology in Castorp's early days at the mountain – he faints, or has a haemorrhage, or a disturbance in appetite, or a fever, and the most curious and droll and nostalgic thoughts and images present themselves to him with lifelike vividness. Physical images – indeed, icons –

in the form of painted pictures, magic lanterns and X-ray plates dominate his thoughts and actions. A whole string of visions or images both praise and bury his poor cousin Joachim; in the eerie light of the fluoroscope Hans peers into Joachim's lighted skeleton, looking ahead metaphorically into Joachim's grave.[16] The grave is prefigured in Joachim's countenance on his deathbed.[17] When Joachim indeed dies, Hans looks into the actual grave. And, sensationally, he sees an apparition of Joachim from *beyond* the grave, conjured forth by presumably foul means at what Mann calls the 'highly questionable' séance towards the novel's end.[18] This string of visions first lures Hans into madness – into being in love with death – and finally shocks him out of it.

One of his more memorable adventures, thought by some to be the book's pinnacle, is also a vision at the very borders of madness and reason, a vision of a (rather hackneyed) Dionysian idyll and a Doric horror of cannibalism, which again, albeit temporarily, shocks him into recovery and the reasoned choosing of life over death.[19]

Vision and morality are memorably tied together. Hans Castorp's world is one in which the *lighting* is crucial, and elaborately staged. Physically it is variously lit by the spooky electrical discharges of the X-ray chamber and the fluoroscope, by the sepulchral light of a séance, by the dazzling blindness of a snowstorm, and by the ghostly illumination of moonlit alpine snowfields. Morally it is lit by the contrasting shades of reason, science, authoritarianism and the occult: everything from the greys of the monk's cell to the ambiguous reds of the boudoir, the bordello and the torture chamber. Within this world, Castorp's madness is an expression of what is intellectually dark and morally questionable; his recovery comes about through shock, and through the ultimately stronger appeal of decency – he morally rejects the necrotic visions of the séance by physically switching on the room lights.[20]

Darkness and creativity

Finally, let us consider the association between creativity and darkness. Of course, Dr. Krokowski would have us begin with the psychoanalytic association between darkness and sexual fecundity. But consider the much wider range of creative acts or impulses across the novel's compass. There are indeed some that are virtuous or benign, but they tend to be presented as futile or misguided – such as Hans Castorp's amateurish attempts at playing the good Samaritan to the dying patients, or his organising a music club for the residents, or Settembrini's construction of an entirely rationalist, so-called 'therapeutic' philosophy of social science, from which a new world order is meant to spring. Much the same might be said of Hofrat Behrens' more imaginative therapeutic *technologies*, such as the 'pleura-shock', the direct electrical stimulation of the lining of the lung cavity, or again of the nature-worship cult ritualised according to Pieter Peeperkorn's gigantic appetite for fine wines and everybody's constant attention. They all get more or less debunked. And more to the point, they tend to be obliterated by altogether darker enterprises: by the manipulative and smutty lecture series by Krokowski; by the dubious pleasures of the bioscope theatre; by the brutalist authority system devised by Naphta; by the occult circle and its séances; and, most importantly, by Hans Castorp's own imaginative excursions into 'being in love with' death and with the knowledge of death.[21]

The earliest stages of this project involve his feverish reconstruction of the emergence of matter from void, of organic life from matter, of consciousness from organic life. This is – or ought to be – the central creative concern of the book. But Mann plays with his materials (and his readers) mischievously. Creation and complexity are cloaked in pollution and impurity, organic growth is represented as pathology. And intriguingly, some of the novel's most startling prose, its most beguiling imagery – even in translation – are reserved for the florid descriptions of the processes of creation as Hans Castorp conjures them. Here is a flavour of what life itself comes to, in this fevered view, variously presented as a

form-preserving instability, a fever of matter, which accompanied the process of ceaseless decay and repair[22]

...that first increase in the density of the spiritual, that pathologically luxuriant morbid growth, produced by the irritant of some unknown infiltration...[23]

the incontinent form of being ... a secret and ardent stirring in the frozen chastity of the universal... conveyed and shaped by the somehow awakened voluptuousness of matter, of the organic, dying-living substance itself, the reeking flesh[24]

And this is explicitly described as the fall. The dark imaginings of Castorp – or of Thomas Mann himself – go on:

The second creation, the birth of the organic out of the inorganic, was only another fatal stage in the progress of the corporeal toward consciousness, just as disease in the organism was an intoxication, a heightening and unlicensed accentuation of its physical state ... life was nothing but the next step on the reckless path of the spirit dishonoured; nothing but the automatic blush of matter roused to sensation and become receptive for that which awaked it.[25]

Stunning images, truly stunning, I think. But what is the message? This descent of the spiritual into the 'reeking flesh' is in effect an upside-down story of *emergence*, of the emergent properties which normally – for us – signal the ascent of the simple into the complex, the sophisticated, the interesting, the meaningful. But if, as does Hans Castorp, you hanker after simplicity, and if you identify purity with non-being, if you are more than half in love with death itself, then of course the creative move towards life, consciousness and meaning is indeed dark and profane. Creation is darkness and profanity. This is a flagrant inversion of our normal expectations, but Thomas Mann is in the inversion business.

Thus, matter emerges from a 'thickening' of the spiritual ether; flesh emerges from matter; the living being emerges from flesh; consciousness and desire emerge from the living being; sensuality and decay emerge from the ambiguities of desire. And from sensuality? Dissolution and, paradoxically, the purity of the grave.

Until the nineteenth century, so Georges Canguilhem tells us, health and disease were seen as locked in combat over the body of Man, in terms reminiscent of the Manichaean combat between good and evil for mastery of the soul.[26] This was a simple enough view – in contrast to the twentieth-century ambiguity of René Leriche's suggestion that disease is less 'a physiology gone wrong than ... a new physiology where many things, tuned in a new key, have unusual resonance'.[27] On the Manichaean view, disease results from the triumph of a kind of evil; but from the pen of Leriche, disease is an altered state of physical matter – in Mann's terms, intoxicated, and hence illicit. Mann refines even this. Life, even matter itself is illicit – the pure disembodied spirit, incarnate, *and hence* dishonoured.

Conclusion

While he is under the Mountain's spell, Hans Castorp himself is minded to oppose the descent of the spirit into life, and to pursue the spiritual purity of death – through adventure, through unguarded, unsupervised intellectual experiment. This is an intoxicating bargain, albeit a bargain with himself as the drafter and the sole signatory. But the madness is highly catching. Are we not ourselves as readers intoxicated by the spin of ideas, the words used, the recklessness of image, of ideas and matter simultaneously emergent from each other and reduced to each other? I know I am. The word 'intoxicated' has an elevating, liberating, even beatific sense for us. I notice, however, that it also means 'poisoned': undeniably, Mann takes roguish delight in the moral ambiguity of his own whirling art, and its part-poisoning, part-liberating effects on his characters – and on us. But why?

To finish – though scarcely to conclude – it is tempting to suppose that Mann is indulging a little guilty speculation about the dark pleasures of literary creation, his own 'sullen art', in Dylan Thomas's words – that alchemy of words whose products are illicit, spellbinding metaphors and images, set to hex and seduce us – deliciously.[28] Mann's capacity for many-layered irony may not be entirely bottomless, but even so we have hardly begun to plumb its depths. The novel is a knowing commentary on its own form, the *Bildungsroman*; it is a silkily self-conscious essay in extended imagery; and every strenuous effort after enlightenment on Hans Castorp's part is cruelly flawed, arousing both our sympathy and our smirks.

It would be mildly perverse, perhaps, but no real surprise, for Mann archly to wring his hands over his own craft in inviting us to compare the darkness of physical creation with 'law-unto-itself' runaway literary invention. If he does, perhaps it is because even the runaway elements in his own invention are so cunningly controlled and choreographed. Admittedly, that is for the *litterati* to judge. My interests are those of the philosopher, but philosophical ideas are sometimes best disclosed (or at any rate illuminated) by the literary imagination. In asking us to think about madness, creativity, the mind, medicine and literature, the editors of this volume are summoning large ideas. The ideas themselves would always summon the philosopher's attention, as compellingly as Hans Castorp was summoned down from the mountain by a military bugle; but the literary imagination allows a silkier, subtler call altogether, and Thomas Mann plays these ideas not upon a bugle but upon Pan's pipes.

Notes

1 Hermann John Weigand, *The Magic Mountain: A Study of Thomas Mann's Novel 'Der Zauerberg'* (Chapel Hill, 1964).

2 Thomas Mann, *The Magic Mountain*, trans. H. T. Lowe-Porter (London, 1999); orig. *Der Zauerberg*, Fischer Verlag, 1924. Page numbers refer to the Vintage edition.

3 Thomas Mann, *Death in Venice and Seven Other Stories*, Vintage International Edition, trans. H. T. Lowe-Porter (New York, 1989), introduction, p. xv.

4 Susan Sontag, *Illness as Metaphor* (New York, 1978).

5 This is Mann's own description of it in a letter on 4th September 1922 to Arthur Schitzler. See Paul Bishop, 'The Intellectual World of Thomas Mann' in *The Cambridge Companion to Thomas Mann*, ed. R. Robertson (Cambridge, 2002), pp. 22–42.

6 Mann, *Magic Mountain*, pp. 218–9

7 T. E. Apter, *Thomas Mann: The Devil's Advocate* (London, 1978); ch. 4.

8 Hans Jonas, 'Against the stream: comments on the definition and re-definition of death' in *Philosophical Essays: From Ancient Creed to Technological Man* (Englewood Cliffs, NJ, 1974), pp. 132–140.

9 Karl Popper, *Conjectures and Refutations* (London, 1963); see especially ch. 1.

10 Thomas Mann, *Doctor Faustus*, transl. H. T. Lowe-Porter (London, 1947), orig. published in German: *Doktor Faustus* (Stockholm, 1947).

11 Martyn Evans, 'The "medical body" as philosophy's arena', *Theoretical Medicine and Bioethics* 2001; 22(1): 17–32.

12 Mann, *Magic Mountain*, p. 217

13 Not all agree – Apter, for instance, appears to find Mann guilty of a confusion in which the physical reduction of, say, emotion to neural events is equated to a

moral or existential reduction. (See Apter, pp. 73–4). My own reading is that Mann allows us to discard the very confusion that he allows some of his characters to commit, not least – to challenge the lesson Apter draws from one particular example – by turning reductionism into arch but palpable buffoonery in the arguments wielded by Hofrat Behrens.

14 Mann, *Magic Mountain*, pp. 257–61.
15 Mann, p. 264.
16 Mann, pp. 217–8.
17 Mann, pp. 534–5.
18 Mann, pp. 680–1.
19 Mann, pp. 490–8.
20 Mann, p. 681.
21 Mann, see especially the chapters 'Research' and 'The dance of death', pp. 267–322.
22 Mann, p. 275.
23 Mann, p. 286.
24 Mann, p. 276.
25 Mann, p. 286.
26 Georges Canguilhem, *On the Normal and the Pathological*, transl. C.R. Fawcett (New York, 1991); originally published as *Le Normal et la Pathologique*, 1966. See especially ch. 1.
27 René Leriche, *Physiologie et pathologie du tissue osseux*, quoted in Canguilhem, *op. cit.*, p. 97.
28 Dylan Thomas, *In my Craft or Sullen Art*, reproduced in Christopher Copeman (ed), *Living and Writing: Dylan Thomas* (London, 1972), p. 1.

Part III
Writing Madness:
Psychoanalysis and Literature

10

Creative Writers and Psychopathology: The Cultural Consolations of 'The Wound and the Bow' Thesis

Patricia Waugh

Edmund Wilson's essay 'Philoctetes: The Wound and the Bow' (1941) has survived as one of the most memorable twentieth-century critical accounts of artistic creativity as an outgrowth of individual psychopathology, of the idea that creative strength is inseparable from disability. Its date of publication coincided with the beginning of a post-Nietzschean revival of the myth of Dionysus, artistic madness as a god-like creativity, or the 'savage god' of Al Alvarez's book of 1971. Nietzsche's version of the myth of Dionysus was pivotal to his critique of scientific rationalism. From *The Birth of Tragedy* until the later works such as *Twilight of the Idols*, Nietzsche reworked the Dionysian legacy of German Romantic thinkers such as Herder and Schelling (for whom Dionysus stood as a symbol of the poetic imagination), into a fully-fledged aesthetic anti-rationalism. Only art might allow a Dionysian dissolution of the self into an harmonious whole reincorporated through the Apollonian discipline of form. In Nietzsche's writings, Dionysus comes to stand as a symbol of psychic renewal through a self-dissolution involving an ecstatic release of the instincts in primordial ritual. Indeed, in the 1886 preface added to *The Birth of Tragedy*, Nietzsche discusses the frenzy and madness of the Dionysian as a neurosis of health, an ecstatic loss of individual self-consciousness and release of repressed desire in communal and ritual ecstasy, a madness which might now constitute the only remaining route back to health. Nietzsche's recapture of the Dionysian was from the earliest writings part of a counter-offensive against the rise of 'theoretic man': the latest version of Socratic rationalism that involved an even more emphatic denial and disavowal of our fundamental primal and erotic energies. His re-reading of the Dionysus myth calls to the original fantasy of the re-incorporation of the savage god, or the stranger within, who must be acknowledged as a prerequisite for psychic renewal. As in Euripides' account, Dionysus is seen to be both master and victim of his own daemonic energies; he is the originator of mind as self-control, but also of madness as a consequence of the refusal and denial of his primal energy in the form of a narrow or instrumental rationality operating through constraint and repression. From the beginning, and certainly in Euripides' account and in Nietzsche's philosophical revival, Dionysus has been invoked as a counterforce against restrictive, instrumental and narrow conceptualisations of reason.

My suggestion in this essay is that the appeal of the myth within modernity has been very much bound up with the encroachment of scientific models of rationality upon areas of culture and human behaviour concerned with values and ends for which science cannot finally legislate. Most recently, this has included the scientific claim to account for mind, consciousness and creativity themselves within the terms of analytical reductionism. The revival of the myth of artistic madness in our own time might be understood as a response to twentieth-century developments in science that have steadily and programmatically reduced a formerly ensouled conception of the human mind to a materialistic model where mind becomes interchangeable with a brain understood as a complex machine. From the behavioural sciences of the twenties to the contemporary fascination with cognitive neuro-psychology, consciousness as intentional subjectivity has been gradually displaced by a third-person account of mind as a kind of algorithmically driven information processor. Post-Cartesian attempts to retain some vestige of ensoulment within a dualistic definition of mind and body have gradually been supplanted by an evolutionary perspective that reduces mind to the materiality of brain, and brain to the digital connections of information technology. As intentionality is gradually decentred, and mind is reconceived within the terms of systems analysis and computer technology, the concept of literary creation, still vital to a modernist aesthetic, has similarly acceded to that of postmodern invention. The revived myth of Dionysus, of the wound of madness as the singing master of the bow, of art as the expression of the tortured or ecstatic soul, can be seen as a consolatory attempt to recover an ensouled idea of the creative human mind in a mechanical and profane world. I will suggest, however, that literary critics and cultural theorists have often embraced the myth rather more enthusiastically and unproblematically than the great modern writers themselves.

In Samuel Beckett's play of 1958, *Endgame*, Hamm remarks to Clov:

> I once knew a madman who thought the end of the world had come. He was a painter – and engraver. I used to go and see him in the asylum. I'd take him by the hand and drag him to the window. Look! There! All that rising corn! And there! Look! The sails of the herring fleet! All that loveliness! He'd snatch away his hand and go back into his corner. Appalled. All he had seen was ashes. (Pause) He alone had been spared. It appears the case is... not so unusual.[1]

The madman in Hamm's story has been spared, he cannot create, for in his madness he sees only the end of creation. All he sees are ashes: no more fertile growth, rising corn, fish in the sea. Beckett pictures madness as a catastrophic loss of the creative power of artistic vision to redeem the suffering of existence. Yet, paradoxically it would seem, madness for Hamm and Clov is a condition devoutly to be desired: the madman who no longer creates has been spared, for in a world of dwindling mythopoeic and theological provenance, tragedy has become this empty 'farce, day after day'. The play presents an image of life where the tragic script which once stood in for destiny has now become ironic and self-reflexive: art can no longer redeem suffering, for the idea of artistic creativity as sacred, a repetition in the material world of the Divine I am, has lost all validity.

Together Clov and Hamm, drained says Hamm by the 'prolonged creative effort', play out, in the eternal recurrence of the theatrical performance, a desire finally to extinguish the ancient ritual of tragedy now turned farce.[2] The modern world has lost the mythopoeic and theological sense of creation, and of art as the redemption of suffering. To know one is trapped in a script, playing an attendant Lord, Hamm, and not even the part of Prince Hamlet; to act one's part, day after day, when there is nothing to be done: such is the ironised tragedy of the modern condition. Beckett seems to enshrine the Nietzschean view of tragedy as the artistic taming of the horrible which rescues us from the absurd and greedy thirst for existence. For Beckett though, in the modern world, we have lost that ensouled idea of creativity as *creation* and are left with merely ingenious and desperate mechanical *invention*, a kind of filibustering against the void, that 'babble, babble', which ends with the feeling, 'ah let's get it over!' Already in 1949, the narrator of Beckett's *The Unnamable* had announced mid-way through the novel:

> I invented it all, in the hope it would console me, help me to go on, allow myself to think of myself as somewhere in a road, moving, between the beginning and the end, but somewhere in the long run making headway. All lies... I have to speak, whatever that means. Having nothing to speak.[3]

Beckett too fears that without the mythopoeic framework of creation, creativity may simply be 'invention', but he refuses to take flight into madness as a consolatory myth. His art is wrought out of a reflection on the problems of living and writing in a culture where invention is becoming all. Beckett's writing is an ethical response to the misery of living in a world no longer sacred. For him, madness offers no consolatory flight from the real, for the problem with the savage god is that his sacred powers are amoral, and like the powers of scientific invention unconstrained by any ethical frame, are as likely to lead to cessation, destruction, violence and killing (the vision of Beckett's madman) as to redemption and joyous liberation.

In the late twentieth century, however, this amoral scientific picture of the world has penetrated more and more into the secret regions of the self and even claims now to explain creativity as simply the firing of neurones and the play of electrical circuits. Such scientific reductionism, of the self to a brain, insidiously confiscates our sense of ourselves as creative and ethical beings. If we are simply chemically determined machines then we can no more feel and be held personally responsible for our lives than if we are mad. Nor can we easily think of ourselves as imaginatively free to shape and create alternative pictures of other possible lives. To think of ourselves as biochemical bodies with biochemical brains is to be as much 'out of our minds' as to be insane. The myth of creative madness has become more seductive in our own culture as an attempt to wrest the dwindling and sacred or even humanist concept of the mystery of selfhood from its ingestion into the scientific machine. A technocratic culture that substitutes a scientistic vocabulary of means for a providential or humanistic discourse of ends diminishes confidence in personal judgement. The pervasive appropriation of mathematical systems analysis, of game theory for example, or theories of rational choice, by political sciences orienting themselves to evolutionary psychological perspectives, both encourages and reflects a contemporary retreat from a conception of the self as an ethical being exercising autonomous choice and creative freedom. The humanist conception of the self as free to choose, free to imagine alternative possibilities, or to achieve existential command over its life and destiny, seems under threat from scientific and postmodern discourses alike. The art and literature of the present overwhelmingly presents the humanist self as vanishing. One might take as an example here the Turner Prize winners of the last few years. Tracy Emin's infamous bed comes immediately to mind. The bed – with its soiled sheets twisted around the evacuated shape of a human form, like the spent cast of some mutilated burrowing creature, the floor around littered with vodka bottles, pills, discarded underwear, used condoms – seemed both testimony to and image of a self pathologically and degradedly out of control, and of art as nihilistically refusing the possibility of formal transcendence. The bed seemed to flaunt the contemporary pathology of the 'borderline personality' as symptomatic of the postmodern condition of 'hyperreality': a condition where art and the self have ceased to exist, not only because their critical transcendence has gone, but also because in a culture of the simulacrum, of endless self-invention and technological reproduction, 'reality itself entirely impregnated with an aesthetic which is inseparable from its own structure, has been confused with its own image'.[4] The bed is certainly the narcissistic exposure of a wound – but is it art, and what has happened to the bow? A year later, the Turner prize was given to another *objet trouvé* – a square electrical light-fitting blinking on and off in a darkened room, an image of the scientific evacuation of human agency favoured in the discourse of the psychopath who describes his act of cold-blooded murder as the switching on and off of an electrical current.

Whilst cultural theorists celebrate spiritual madness as they revive the savage god Dionysus, bio-medical science reduces mental illness to chemical imbalances and faulty wiring in the brain: as if the mind were a kind of television set subject to electrical interference and faulty reception, but available for a quick technical fix, a new socket, or an improved circuit. Patricia Churchland, eminent American neuro-philosopher, argues, for example, that

> what is so exciting is that philosophical questions raised by the Greeks are coming within the province of science. We now have an enormous opportunity...to understand and to treat such devastating malfunctions as depression, drug addiction and schizophrenia.[5]

This is the brave new world of the brain sciences: 'Our world has chosen machinery and medicine and happiness' says the world-controller, Mustapha Mond, in Huxley's novel of 1931.[6] As in our own brave new world, its cultural rebel, the savage John, embraces madness as the only sacred alternative: he crucifies himself in a Dionysian frenzy, quoting Shakespeare to the very last. Shakespeare also, of course, famously entertained the Dionysian myth in *A Midsummer Night's Dream*. Theseus observes the similarities between the lover, the lunatic and the poet. All are possessed by frenzied visions, fantasies, but the creativity of the poet is presented as qualitatively different. In all three, 'imagination bodies forth / The forms of things unknown', but 'the poet's pen / Turns them to shapes, and gives to airy nothing / A local habitation and a name'.[7] Poetry is still for Shakespeare that divinised act where, in a 'fine frenzy', chaos is rent to give shape and form to new worlds. In the twentieth century it is the unconscious of psychoanalysis, or so it seems, which has carried the divine metaphor of inspiration, of creation as primordial darkness breaking into light. But for us, Daybreak is imaged as a reverse journey, not shape out of chaos, but the flight from a repressive scientific rationality and descent into the chaos of madness as the recovery of the lost seat of the soul. Our cultural theorists have briefed us for a descent into hell.

The myth has been powerful throughout the century: from Nietzsche to Freud to the counter-cultural offensives of R. D. Laing and the seductions of Alvarez's savage god to a final florescence in postmodernism and much contemporary feminism. Hysteria is celebrated as a discourse of feminine resistance to the Law; the Lacanian Imaginary as a decentring, dissolution and fragmentation of the symbolic order; Deleuzian 'schizanalysis' as the political breaking of the iron cage of rationality. In each of these discourses, madness becomes the mode of Daybreak, the mode in which creativity might be salvaged in the violent destruction of those scientific chains that bind us in an iron cage of reason. I want to suggest though that the myth may not be so conducive to creativity and self-liberation as its intellectual expositors claim. Apparently offering consolation in the form of resistance to an instrumental rationality, it also shares some of the features of what it claims to oppose. The most powerfully insidious of these is a shared model of reason. If post-Cartesian method, analytic reductionism, scientific rationality, are assumed to be all that reason might be, then madness, 'going out of your mind', 'losing your reason', 'taking leave of your sense' or being 'off your head', seem the only escape from the cage. But the desired dissolution of subjectivity into the 'desiring machine' of postmodern philosophy has the same cultural effect as the destruction of intentionality by that biological computing machine, the algorithmically emergent brain of modern biological science. Both evacuate belief and trust in the self as free to shape its world and to make ethical choices.

The revival of Dionysus in the madness-as-liberation myth achieved its most ecstatic recovery in the counter-culture and anti-psychiatry movements of the sixties, but has lived on to inhabit the assumptions of much postmodern writing. But let us pause for a moment and compare Laing's account of Dionysus with his embodiment in the most famous extant account from the Greek world – Euripides' play *The Bacchae*. For Laing, insanity is not an abandonment of the real but an intelligible attempt to achieve ontological security in a violent and competitive society. In a Nietzschean twist, a revaluation of values that situates the self beyond good and evil, the madman becomes the image of authentic selfhood: madness is a refusal of the slave morality whose violence destroys those ascetic fictions which compel our conformity through internalised guilt and shame. Laing's book *The Politics of Experience* of 1967 is pervaded with the metaphor of the Dionysian as daybreak, of madness as breakthrough, liberation and renewal, as much as breakdown, enslavement and existential death. He argues that 'true sanity entails in one way or another the dissolution of the normal ego, that false self competently adjusted to our alienated social reality; the emergence of the inner archetypal mediators of divine power, and through this death a rebirth, and the eventual re-establishment of a new kind of ego-functioning, the ego now being the servant of the divine, no longer its betrayer'.[8] At first glance, Euripides' play seems to bear out Laing's Nietzschean account of the Dionysian. Dionysus comes to Thebes as a stranger, disguised as an adolescent boy, proclaiming at the start of the play: 'I am come! – a god standing on ground / Where I was born in Thebes / Lightning ripped me from the pregnant body of Semele / That blast of flame was my midwife'.[9] In the play, those who most fervently employ their cunning and reason to resist him are either driven completely mad or die a violent death. Pentheus, the rationalist, whose will-to-knowledge is presented as a ruthless will-to-power, can see that in his obsession with hunting down Dionysus, he is 'hopelessly entangled with this stranger'. He is unable to acknowledge the erotic quality of the entanglement and therefore backs away disgustedly from Dionysus's seductive power: 'don't smear your craziness off onto me'.[10] The play ends with his violent dismemberment. Tiresias, himself a convert to the Dionysian mysteries, looks on throughout commentating on events. Like Laing, he too appears to reverse the images of madness and sanity, accusing Pentheus of 'sick fantasies' and of suffering from a 'raging brain fever' for denying the god. It is difficult now not to read the play psychoanalytically, (as a parable of the violent consequences if we try to simply repress or shut out our irrational impulses), with the unconscious viewed as the savage god, the stranger within, who will liberate us from the iron cage of reason. Unlike Laing's work, however, Euripides' play contains more than one model of reason. Those, like Pentheus, who assume rationality in the mode of technocratic control, are destroyed; more significantly, however, so are those who simply give themselves up entirely to the Laingian style self-dissolution of the Bacchanalian frenzy. It is Tiresias who sees that it is the manner of our reception of the god that matters, and that depends on our already-formed ethical dispositions. Tiresias is the vehicle for this under-standing of reason: 'even at the peak of Bacchic abandon', he says, 'a chaste woman remains perfectly chaste'.[11] Reason conceived not as technocratic control but as an ethical disposition, a cultivation and care of the self, incorporates but is not destroyed by the god. True sanity, in contradistinc-tion to the Laingian interpretation, is an acknowlegement and reception of the god within the bounds of reason exercised as an ethical agency. It is interesting, of course, that Foucault himself began to turn towards this idea in his late writings shortly before his death.

Whether it is imposed as an 'objective' bio-medical label or willingly embraced as a subjective mode of liberation, insanity places the madman outside the realm of ethical responsibility – legally, the mad are not held responsible for their actions. The imposed label 'mad' confiscates our sover-eign subjectivity but so does its willed or willing embrace. Contemporary science is also ever busy confiscating our responsibility, reducing our confidence in ourselves as beings with free will and choice by constructing endless pathological syndromes for us – in a recent court action, for example, the defense lawyer for a mass murderer used the insanity plea in describing his client as suffering from 'urban survival syndrome'. It was his syndrome not himself responsible. We are now told that there is a gene for violence. Edmund in Shakespeare's *King Lear* reflects that it is the 'excellent foppery' of his age that 'when we are sick in fortune... we make guilty of our disasters the sun, the moon, and stars, as if we were villains on neces-sity, fools by heavenly compulsion'.[12] It seems that we now prefer that fool-ishness and villainy are written into our genes rather than the stars, that our disposition and ethos are carried by the 'necessary' logic of (ultra-Darwinist) natural selection. The tendency surely reflects a desire for certainty; that reason conceived as scientific method might deliver ends and purposes as well as means, offering a shortcut to ethical judgement and the determination of values. Iris Murdoch once observed that human beings are creatures who make pictures of themselves and try to live in accord with such pictures. Public mediations of the contemporary biological sciences have been preoccupied with the construction of a picture of the human as a 'lumbering robot' (in Dawkins' infamous phrase), a kind of driverless juggernaut delivering the eternally self-replicating 'selfish genes' that will build our progeny. We are, he insists in a recent book, a 'secondary derived phenomenon, cobbled together as a consequence of fundamentally separate, warring agents'.[13] Mad or genetically engineered by nature, however, we need not be held or feel responsible for our actions. The genes, says E. O. Wilson, in his recent book *Consilience*, have culture on a leash and, by a process of analytical reduction, the scientist may deliver up knowledge of those very material foundations which finally determine our cultural ends and purposes.[14] The human self as a creative and intentional agent is eliminated and mind once again reduced to the algorithmic functioning of the processes of natural selection hard-wired into our neuronal circuits.

Richard Dawkins, like the philosopher of science Daniel Dennett, insists on an account of mind as an emergent property of genetic coding, built by cranes and disseminated by memes, rather than operating through intentionality and accounted for through philosophically idealist 'skyhooks'. Evolutionary psychologists are even more ambitious in their destruction of our ethical selves. Not content with mechanical invention, they want to capture the myth of creation too. Where Beckett proposes a valedictory lament for the dying in our culture of that ancient mythopoeic and theological frame which valued the artistic imagination, the scientist will now become the priest and scribe of the Divine I am. Matt Ridley's book *Genome* opens in a mocking parody of Genesis:

> In the beginning was the word. The word proselytised the sea with its message, copying itself unceasingly and forever. The word discovered how to rearrange chemicals so as to capture little eddies in the stream of entropy and make them live...became sufficiently ingenious to build a porridgy contraption called a human brain that could discover and be aware of the word itself.[15]

The 'word', of course, is the code of DNA: Logos, prime-mover, architect and master-builder. The human self hovers between machine and abstract information system; DNA takes on all the attributes of human agency in its building and binding, mobilising and penetrating, communication and combining. As in the currently fashionable cultural theories which celebrate subjective dissolution with post-Dionysian enthusiasm, the text (whether the code of DNA as a writing which writes or the endless agon of the postmodern 'material' signifier) becomes more real than the real; the body is writing, and, in both accounts, the self as intentional agent, ethical being, human creature with free will and control over its circumstances, is evacuated. Mind, belief and intentionality are shredded in the eliminative machines of neuro-scientific and postmodern reductionism.

How does Freudian psychoanalysis fit into this proposed cultural narrative? I want to consider this by examining in more detail Wilson's essay, 'Philoctetes: The Wound and the Bow'. Just as Laing at the start of the sixties began his 'anti-psychiatry' reading of *The Bacchae*, Wilson at the start of the forties had offered a Freudian reading of Sophocles' play *Philoctetes*. His essay interprets the play as a parable of the rise of civilisation out of our discontents; as a plea for the need to recognise therefore that though art is rooted in psychopatholgy, the artist is the sacred pariah we cannot do without. The play tells the story of the Greek Philoctetes who, armed with his magical and invincible bow, a gift from Heracles, is part of a military expedition to Troy, but on the journey is bitten by a venomous snake. The wound will not heal and begins to supurate odoriferously. Philoctetes' companions are sickened and disgusted by the obnoxious flux and his agonised 'frantic wailing'. They abandon him on the Isle of Lemnos, condemning him to exile. Ten years later they return, led by Odysseus who, convinced that the Greeks cannot prevail over the Trojans without the magical bow, has conceived a plot to trick Philoctetes into giving up his beloved weapon. They first discover his vacated bed, a pile of leaves in a cave, littered with blood-stained rags and other evidence that the wound has never healed, and they come to find Philoctetes now 'near out of his mind' and crazed with pain. 'What is the power of the play'? asks Wilson. 'Philoctetes remains in our mind, and his incurable wound and invincible bow recur to us with a special insistence. But what is it they mean? How is it possible for Sophocles to make us accept them so naturally? Why do we enter with scarcely a stumble into the situation of people who are preoccupied with a snakebite that lasts for ever and a weapon that cannot fail?'[16] André Gide had rewritten the play for his own time and presented Philoctetes explaining to Neoptolamus, the boy who is to carry out Odysseus's trickery, that he has mastered his pain through language, for 'if the phrase was very beautiful...I was by so much consoled... I came to understand that words inevitably become more beautiful from the moment they are no longer put together in response to the demands of others'.[17] Gide's Philoctetes is explicitly the artist as outcast. Wilson adds the sacred touch by effectively if implicitly treating Sophocles' play as a theodicy that offers up creativity as the justification for suffering. The Greeks know they cannot win the Trojan War without the bow, but they have to come to recognise too that 'they cannot have the irresistible weapon without its loathsome owner, who upsets the processes of normal life by his curses and his cries'.[18] Wilson's assumptions, of course, reiterate the Freudian claim that 'the essential *ars poetica* involves the technique of overcoming the feeling of repulsion in us when we encounter the fantasies and psychopathology of the artist out of which the work necessarily arises'.[19] Beautiful phrases redeem suffering. Wilson turns to psychoanalysis as a discourse which might justify art as a powerful force for cultural healing and transcendence, but without denying either its unique formal autonomy or its daemonic galvanisation in the crucible of individual pain and suffering.

Wilson's reading, like Laing's version of Dionysus, is powerful but selective and ahistorical. What is occluded is surely the crucial moment in the play: the moment when Neoptolemus takes pity on Philoctetes by seeing him face to face as a fellow human being and not simply as an incurable medical case to be shut away out of sight. Neoptolemus heroically opens himself to the ethical demand, decides to refuse to be the agent of Odysseus's trickery, and becomes an ethical agent himself. He reveals to Philoctetes the deception, and reveals to himself the emptiness of Odysseus's supposed 'noble lie'. Having earlier seized the bow he gives it back even though he also knows that this is likely to bring about his own death. He does not simply give back the bow because he sees that it is useless without its rightful owner (Wilson's psychoanalytic reading), he gives it back because he sees that it is morally wrong to seize the bow through a deception practised on an ill and suffering man. Because of Neoptolemus's honesty, Philoctetes is able to regain his own trust in humanity and to give up his desire for revenge. The play is about the self-confidence and honesty required for trust, as much as it is a parable of the artist as sacred pariah. The play addresses the ethical imperative to, in T. S. Eliot's formulation, 'give, sympathise and control', and suggests there can be neither art nor the proper art of living unless ethical reason, which is wisdom, helps to shape the terms of our mortal condition, the wound of living.

But the more internalised the modern paradigm of a purely scientific reason becomes for us, the more we seem only able to envisage our opposition to and liberation from it in the terms of creative madness or the frenzy of the Dionysian. I want to look now at the more general contribution of Freudianism to these assumptions, by approaching Freud's work through another American critic of the mid-century, Lionel Trilling, for whom Freudian psychoanalysis represented a means of strengthening the idea of the autonomy of the liberal self in an increasingly rationalised and controlling society (the winds of the Cold War, of American corporatism and Soviet communism were blowing sharply at Trilling's back when he discovered psychoanalysis). Trilling reads Freudian psychoanalysis as a humanist account that makes poetry indigenous to the human mind in its description of the unconscious operating through a language of displacement (metonymy), condensation (metaphor), and symbolisation. Certainly, psychoanalysis appears to be more humanistic in its account of the mind and of psychopathology than our contemporary brain sciences, and for that reason has survived and flourished in literary criticism and disappeared almost entirely from the discipline of psychology. Again though, it is possible to read the Freudian account of mind as an earlier twentieth-century moment of 'epic science' which also claimed to offer an account of culture premised on a bedrock of biological explanation.

The terms of his praise for Freud might give us pause for further reflection on Trilling's interpretation of the Freudian account of mind. In a late book of 1972, *Sincerity and Authenticity*, Trilling notes that 'Freud in insisting upon the essential unmitigability of the human condition as determined by the nature of the mind, had the intention of sustaining the authenticity of human existence that formerly had been ratified by God...Like the Book of Job [Freud's work] propounds and accepts the mystery and naturalism of suffering'.[20] Earlier, in his book *Beyond Culture*, published in 1965, Trilling observes that 'somewhere in the child, somewhere in the adult, there is a hard irreducible stubborn core of biological urgency ... that culture cannot reach and that reserves the right... to judge the culture and to resist and revise it... We cannot name the work of any great writer of the modern period whose work has not in some way...expressed the bitterness of his discontent with civilisation, who has not said the self made greater legitimate clams than the culture could hope to satisfy...We can speak no greater praise of Freud than to say that he placed this idea at the very centre of his thought'.[21] The reference to the Book of Job suggests that Trilling, like Wilson before him, wants to read psychoanalysis as a theodicy. But the quotation from *Beyond Culture* suggests that it would be more accurate to view Trilling's view of Freud as the constructor of a biodicy.

The Freudian account of mind is a parable of creation: of the emergence of order (thinking, rationality) out of the chaos of sensation and the biological drives. As in earlier cosmologies, the emergence of order, the order of the self, involves a painful tearing, a separation, like Dionysus ripped from Semele's womb, and may give rise to an oceanic longing to dissolve back into primordial matter (the death-drive) or to find release in frenzy or escape into neurosis or psychosis. Art functions here as a more desirable substitute, a mode of reparation through sublimation of conflict and division. The idea of artistic creativity gives to the Freudian account the transferred resonance of the Greek and Judaeo-Christian theodicy, for art, creativity, is the place in this life, this biological existence, where in the end, we find our happiness or not at all. In the absence of an operative *theos*, the biological drives that are the origin of the unconscious now become the source and bedrock of our cultural redemption, our modern version of divine inspiration. But Freud, the positivist scientist, needs biology as the bedrock of his account of mind and culture, as much as Freud, the thaumaturgist, needs to transfer into biology and via art the idea of the soul and the mysteries of mythopoeic and theological creation. If creative writers perform the unconscious then Freud will 'excavate' (a favourite metaphor of his) down to its biological bedrock and name it as grammarian of the palimpsest of the human soul. Just as Plato accuses the rhapsode of epistemological occlusion – that unlike the philosopher he cannot stand outside of the artistic performance and rationally know and name what he knows, so too Freud, as crypto-biologist, claims epistemological superiority as modern scientist of the soul who will map and chart its strange seas.

Perhaps both Plato and Freud suffered from poetry-envy. Certainly they both show a profound ambivalence towards poetic art, a need for it and a need to master and control it. At times, creative writers are seen to 'know a whole host of things between heaven and earth of which our philosophy has not let us dream' though, adds Freud, signalling his view of the future role of psychoanalysis, 'they draw on sources which have not yet opened up for science'. But Freud is also openly reductive, seeing the artist as driven by 'excessively powerful instinctual needs. He desires to win honour, power, wealth, fame and the love of women, but he lacks the means for achieving these satisfactions. Consequently, like any other unsatisfied man, he turns away from reality and transfers all his interest, and his libido too, to the wishful construction of his life of phantasy, whence the path might lead to neurosis'.[22] Art is reduced to the favourite example of contemporary evolutionary psychologists, the peacock's tail, a mode of display and glamour whose apparent uselessness is actually a mark of quality, of luxurious excess which guarantees sexual selection. Like Dionysus, with his 'soft unmuscular body' and pubescent girlishness, Freud's artist too is an adolescent, sexually ambiguous and neurotic, but who gains power, sexual identity, and cultural status by seducing us into his fantasy life. But whereas Euripides places Dionysus in the frame of ethical reason, Freud's artist will be placed in the frame of modern science. The artist plays out his hysterical symptoms through the body of his work and Freud, like the geneticists and psychoanalytic critics of our own time, will decipher the text of his soul.

The immediate appeal of Freudianism was that it seemed to offer a more complex and humanistic and ensouled idea of the mind than the prevailing psychiatric Darwinism of doctors such as Henry Maudsley and George Savage (one of Virginia Woolf's doctors and the model for Sir William Bradshaw in *Mrs Dalloway*). Such accounts presented mental illness as a consequence of 'degeneration', of nervous heredity, and tended also to explain artistic genius as arising from a disordered physiology. But the

Freudian account makes many of the same assumptions. In Max Nordau's immensely popular book of 1895, *Degeneration*, he explains that:

> Degenerates are not always criminals, prostitutes, anarchists and pro-
> nounced lunatics; they are often authors and artists. These, however,
> manifest the same mental characteristics, and for the most part the same
> somatic features as the above-mentioned anthropological family, who
> satisfy their unhealthy impulses with the knife of the assassin or the
> bomb of the dynamiter, instead of with pen and pencil.[23]

Freud works with similar assumptions; he simply removes the overtly moralising cast of the discourse.

Not surprisingly, most of the great modern writers saw through the myth and struggled to develop alternatives both to the irrationalist myth of creative madness and to the scientific appropriation of the concept of reason. Joseph Conrad's *The Secret Agent* of 1907, for example, certainly presents his anarchists and dynamitists as degenerates but in order to deconstruct the medicalisation of degeneration itself as the real degeneracy: the desire of a scientised culture to substitute a medical label for the evasion of personal responsibility (secret agency) understood as the hard work of looking 'deeply into things', knowing and controlling one's own actions. Though recognising the symbolic value of exploding the Greenwich Observatory as an icon of scientific fetishisation, each of the anarchists exposes his own version of the fetish: dialectical materialism, bio-medical theory, technocratic infatuation. Joyce's Stephen Daedalus is initially seduced by the sacred connotations of Dionysian creativity calling to him as liberation from the dull gross voice of the world of duties and despair, but in the moment of ecstatic vision on the sand he can only cry out inchoately ('no words passed his lips') like a hawk or an eagle, and like Philoctetes nursing his wound, must patiently and reflectively learn that aesthetic craft of words which will allow his bow to sing. So too, Eliot's 'individual talent' does not arise spontaneously like Jung's out of a Lamarckian collective unconscious, but must be actively shaped through the strenuous task of recovering a tradition and submitting to the 'intolerable wrestle with words' which is the making of the poem. It is perhaps in the writing of Virginia Woolf, of all the moderns, however, that the concepts of mind, madness, creativity and literature are most explicitly engaged in ways that suggest both the seductive call of dissolution for the creative writer, and an equally powerful imperative to transcend and control such impulses.

Woolf was herself diagnosed as mad and subjected to a variety of psychiatric treatments. Even with two trained Freudian analysts in her immediate family, though, she continually resisted analysis, insisting that she had achieved through her writing what psychoanalysts did for their patients. In a review of 1920, 'Freudian Fiction', she rejects psychoanalysis as a kind of pseudo-science: 'Yes, says the scientific side of the brain, that... explains a great deal. No, says the artistic side of the brain, that is dull and has no human significance'.[24] We won't discover the mind in Harley Street, she wryly noted in her diary after managing to resist the psychiatric Darwinist Sir George Savage's proposal to extract her teeth in order to cure her auditory hallucinations. But she experienced her illnesses (which would probably be diagnosed now as bipolar disorder) as much physically as mentally. The purely (philosophically) idealist account of the mind seemed to her as evasive in its mysticism as the purely scientific account was reductionist in its materialism. One of the most interesting meditations on the problem is an essay written by Woolf in 1926, 'On Being Ill', which begins by noting 'how tremendous the spiritual changes that it brings... when the lights of health go down', for as 'the body smashes itself to smithereens...the soul (it is said) escapes'.[25] The qualification implied in parentheses is significant – no psychoanalytic wound and bow thesis here – yet, she goes on to suggest, without the 'courage of a lion-tamer' or a 'robust philosophy', 'this miracle, pain, will soon make us taper into mysticism, or rise with rapid beats of the wings, into the raptures of transcendentalism'.[26] What medical science will name with the vocabulary of pathology, the writer must try to convey as an experience. We need a new language, she says 'more primitive, more sensual, more obscene'.[27] Pain seems to defy translation into words, yet as for Philoctetes, without the recognition achieved through its communication, we become exiles within ourselves. Pain forces us to acknowledge, she says at the end of the essay, the isolation of the soul, that 'there is a virgin forest in each; a snowfield where even the print of bird's feet is unknown'. Yet the bleaching out of meaning that occurs in the experience of suffering, the emptying out of denotative sense, the white of the snowfield, also allows the materiality of language, its poetry even, to seize our senses: 'in health meaning has encroached upon sound', but in illness 'words give out their scent and distill their flavour'.[28] For Woolf, the wound is an aspect of the bow, and she did believe that there was something mystical about her own madnesses – that they served her for religion – but madness is insufficient in itself to account for the bow. The phrase 'tapering into mysticism' is heavily ironic: to make art also requires the courage of the lion-tamer, the robust philosophy, what she several times refers to as 'backbone', a word physical, formal and moral in its connotations.

All of Woolf's writing expresses this desire to reach beyond that 'talk' which is speech without form. In an essay called 'Life and the Novelist' of 1927, she dismisses three-quarters of the fiction of her day as writing 'soft and shapeless with words... upon real lips' and giving no relief from the 'swarm and confusion of life'. The art of writing must have 'backbone', 'something compelling words to shape' and a novel should be 'like a Chinese coat able to stand by itself'.[29] In Woolf's 1927 novel *To the Lighthouse*, Lily Briscoe, the artist, experiences a kind of dissolution of self, a negation of ego as she begins the final work of completing her painting, 'losing her name, her personality', but this is not negation in the Freudian sense of a turning away from the real and into the life of fantasy or Dionysian frenzy, it is a disciplining of self into detachment.[30] Negation in art is shown to involve a capacity to stand back from ordinary engagement with the world and, through the controlled renunciation of ego, to reach beyond 'ordinary perception', customary talk, those screens of 'common sense' that shut us up in rooms and shut us out from each other. For Lily Briscoe, the painter, it involves the strenuous effort to discover that back-bone or 'design' which compels to shape words which paradoxically can then be more 'more primitive, more sensuous, more obscene'. Again, in her essay 'The Narrow Bridge of Art', Woolf describes the artistic process in similar terms: 'there emerges from the mist something stark, something for-midable and enduring, the bone and substance upon which our rush of indiscriminating emotion was founded'.[31] Notice how often her language mixes bodily synechdoches – skeleton, bone, backbone – with the language of emotion; and how often she concretises mind as a room or a virgin snowfield where not even the print of a bird's foot may be seen. Woolf struggles to discover a means through poetic language to overcome the dualism of mind and body but without either collapsing mind into the reductionist labelling of bio-medical discourse and positivist science, or tapering off into idealism or irrationalist mysticism that she said 'wraps the world around in cotton wool'.[32] Bertrand Russell, a philosopher who influenced the thought of Bloomsbury, likewise laughed at the physical reductionism of the psychoanalytic unconscious as a picture of a kind of 'chained prisoner in a dungeon hurling itself at the walls with strange groans and atavistic lusts'.[33] He described his 1923 book *The Analysis of Mind* as an attempt to 'persuade you that matter is not so material and mind not so mental as is generally supposed. When we are speaking of matter, it will seem as if we were inclining to idealism; when we are speak-ing of mind, it will seem as if we are inclining to materialism. Neither is the truth'.[34] In *Mrs Dalloway*, written two years later, Woolf tried to articulate this idea through what she described as a study of insanity and sanity seen side by side. Septimus Smith, back from the war, one of Wilfred Owen's men whose minds the Dead have ravaged, is suffering from shellshock after seeing his friend Evans killed. Shellshock was a condition as likely to produce hysterical conversion symptoms in the body – paralysis, mutism – as that mental derangement which Septimus experiences as an inability to feel. He has felt too much and now cannot 'feel' that he even exists, but then he has been drilled into a war regime which requires absence of 'feeling' as the mark of sanity, and into a social system where the absence of feeling is manliness. His madness is diagnosed by the psychiatrist Bradshaw as losing his sense of proportion. Septimus cannot feel himself in his own body but can experience himself as part of the trees and believes that his soul has taken flight and mystically dissolved into the universe. Clarissa has stayed sane by shutting out passion, by containing the haunting voices of the past inside her head, by resisting the 'violators of the soul', but she too suffers (literally) from a defective heart and a problem of feeling; she too experiences herself as an absence at the core. Where Septimus feels himself dissolved out into the universe, Clarissa carries a sense of not having 'something central which permeated'.[35] Like Septimus too, she feels herself invisible, Mrs Richard Dalloway, M.P.'s wife and socialite, and now middle-aged and menopausal, giving herself only as the party hostess, and afterwards withdrawing safely into her chaste and narrow room. The novel reaches towards its conclusion as Clarissa at her party hears of Septimus's suicide. The reader has already learned of the suicide, the moment when Septimus flings himself out of the window, crying of his life, himself, 'I'll give it you'.[36] Similarly, as Clarissa hears the mention of his death in the midst of her party, she senses her own life as an emptying of the soul, not as a gift, however, but herself 'let drop every day in corruption, lies, chatter'.[37] Septimus's death she understands then as 'an attempt to communicate'. Like Neoptolemus with Philoctetes, she listens to Septimus's voice 'bodied forth' in her own internal dialogue – the voices in her head – and though it is too late to minister to his soul, she can minister to her own. In the revelatory moment of recognition and identification, she understands the failings of her own soul, its trickeries and lies, refracted back in the image of his demise. With her 'defective heart', she has controlled but not sympathised, not given. Septimus is mad because he has given, has sympathised, but has been controlled and has lost control. Septimus wanted to be a poet, idolised Keats, but can no longer create, can only doodle nonsense. He has evaded the scientific reductionisms of the psychiatric profession, but only at the price of a dissolution of selfhood which finally destroys him. For Woolf sees that for the bow to redeem the wound, the artist must give, sympathise *and* control. Reason conceived on the model of 'a sense of proportion' is the modern equivalent of Pentheus's technocratic control: it is the other face of madness. Reason conceived as an ethical openness to the other (within and without) is the equivalent of the true creative artist's capacity to surrender the self as a gift, but within the terms of a formal design which expresses that self in a more complete, if still ever incomplete, mode.

Notes

1 Samuel Beckett, *Endgame* (London, 1964), p. 32.
2 Beckett, *Endgame*, pp. 26, 41.
3 Samuel Beckett, *The Unnammable* (London, 1959), p. 316.
4 Jean Baudrillard, *Simulations* (New York, 1983), pp. 151–2.
5 Patricia Churchland, 'Glimpses of the mind', *Time Magazine*, July 17, 1995, p. 44.
6 Aldous Huxley, *Brave New World* (Harmondsworth, 1955), p. 183.

7 William Shakespeare, *A Midsummer Night's Dream*, in *The Complete Works*, ed. Stanley Wells and Gary Taylor (Oxford, 1988) V, i, 12–17.

8 R. D. Laing, *The Divided Self* (Harmondsworth, 1971), pp. 144–5.

9 Euripides, *The Bacchae*, trans. Robert Bagg (New York, 1990), p. 369.

10 Euripides, p. 383.

11 Euripides, p. 382.

12 Shakespeare, *The Tragedy of King Lear*, in *Complete Works*, I, ii, 116–18.

13 Richard Dawkins, *Unweaving the Rainbow: Science, Delusion and the Capacity for Wonder* (London, 1998), p. 308.

14 E. O. Wilson, *Consilience: The Unity of Knowledge* (London, 1998).

15 Matt Ridley, *Genome* (London, 1999), p. 11.

16 Edmund Wilson, *The Wound and the Bow* (London, 1961), pp. 246–7.

17 Wilson, p. 259.

18 Wilson, p. 264.

19 Sigmund Freud, 'Creative writers and daydreaming', in *The Standard Edition of the Complete Psychological Works of Sigmund Freud*, ed. and trans. James Strachey et al., 24 vols (London, 1953–74), vol. 9, repr. in David Lodge, ed., *Twentieth-Century Literary Criticism* (London, 1988), p. 42.

20 Lionel Trilling, *Sincerity and Authenticity* (Oxford, 1972), p. 156.

21 Trilling, *Beyond Culture* (Harmondsworth, 1967), p. 107.

22 Sigmund Freud, 'Delusions and dreams in Jensen's Gradiva', in *Standard Edition*, vol. 9, p. 8.

23 Max Nordau, *Degeneration* (London, 1895), preface.

24 Virginia Woolf, 'Freudian Fiction', in *The Essays of Virginia Woolf*, ed. Andrew McNeillie, vol. 3 (London, 1986), p. 197.

25 Virginia Woolf, 'On Being Ill', in *The Crowded Dance of Modern Life*, ed. Rachel Bowlby (Harmondsworth, 1993), p. 43.

26 Woolf, 'On Being Ill', p. 44.

27 Woolf, 'On Being Ill', p. 45

28 Woolf, 'On Being Ill', p. 46.

29 Virginia Woolf, 'Life and the Novelist', in *Granite and Rainbow* (London, 1958), p. 42.

30 Virginia Woolf, *To The Lighthouse* (London, 1927), p. 246.

31 Virginia Woolf, 'The Narrow Bridge of Art', in *Granite and Rainbow*, p. 23.

32 Virginia Woolf, in *The Captain's Deathbed and Other Essays* (New York, 1950), p. 86.

33 Bertrand Russell, *The Analysis of Mind* (London, 1995), p. 38.

34 Russell, p. 36.

35 Virginia Woolf, *Mrs Dalloway* (Harmondsworth, 1964), p. 36.

36 Woolf, *Mrs Dalloway*, p. 165.

37 Woolf, *Mrs Dalloway*, p. 204.

11
The Myth of the Artist

Al Alvarez

I'm going to talk about a period in the 1960s and '70s when art and mental disturbance seemed closely linked, and I want to begin with a fragment of partial and potted literary history. In the first quarter of the twentieth century, the great period of experimental Modernism, 'advanced' literary people were arguing that Romanticism was finally dead and a new period of Classicism had begun. T. E. Hulme wrote a brilliant essay on the theme that influenced T. S. Eliot so profoundly that he called Hulme, who wrote little and died young, 'the forerunner of a new attitude of mind, which should be called the twentieth century mind'.[1] Hulme dismissed Romanticism as 'spilt religion' because it yearned for the infinite, distrusted the intellect and paid rather cursory attention to detail.[2] In contrast, Classicism was the opposite of all that; it implied, among other things, impersonality, intelligence, lucidity, control. In other words, Modernism was an impatient reaction against Romantic self-indulgence and mindlessness; the artists were surfeited with wine and roses and atmosphere; it was time for an altogether more strenuous and unforgiving style.

Just how powerful and reasonable their case was becomes clear if you compare a poem by, say, Swinburne – full of verbal colour and rhythmic excitement, but with little to say and vague as to how the pieces fit together – with the deliberately fragmented and allusive style of *The Waste Land*, where a great deal is implied and very little stated outright. It becomes even more powerful if you compare the Swinburne with Eliot's notes to *The Waste Land,* which was where the real polemics were; they implied that the reader should have read not just the classics in several languages but also books which had no obvious connection with poetry, like Frazer's *Golden Bough*, F. H. Bradley's *Appearance and Reality*, Jessie Weston's *From Ritual to Romance*, and the *Handbook of Birds of Eastern North America*; they should also be able to work out references, follow an argument, and leap semantic gaps. (My own belief is that the notes were a smokescreen; if you read the poem itself, you got an utterly different impression: that of a precise, delicate and not particularly defended portrait of a man having a nervous breakdown. But that was not a topic Eliot wished to draw attention to and the notes were a way of confusing the issue. They were also a way of padding out a relatively short poem into something that could be published as a book.)

As it turned out, Eliot, Hulme and the others were not wrong about Classicism, they were simply optimistic. History was not on their side. Throughout the last century every enlightened step forward – in science, technology, social justice, the elimination of poverty, and so on – was counter-balanced by crazed eruptions of irrationality and barbarism: World Wars, genocide, terrorism and endemic totalitarianism, symbolised most clearly and brutally by that peculiarly twentieth-century innovation, the death camp, where the technology was used to set up factories for the efficient production of corpses. In the face of all that, it became increasingly difficult to believe in the supremacy of order and sweet reason. Naturally, it took time for all that to sink in, but by the end of the 1950s something more complex and less clear-cut seemed to be demanded.

Thirty years ago, in a book called *The Savage God*, I tried to suggest what that something might be. I called it Extremist art, by which I meant an art which goes out along that friable edge between the tolerable and intolerable, yet does so with all the discipline and clarity and attention to detail Eliot implied when he talked of Classicism. Where the Extremists – Robert Lowell, John Berryman and Sylvia Plath, above all – parted company with Eliot was not in his devotion to the stern discipline of art but in his doctrine of impersonality – 'an escape from personality', he called it.[3] Extremist artists – the Abstract Expressionist painters as well as the poets – deliberately used their chaotic personal lives – Lowell was a manic depressive, Berryman and Jackson Pollock were alcoholics, Plath and Rothko were depressed to the point of psychosis – in order to set up a mirror to the chaos out there in the world. In other words, Extremism was an existentialist art form, one in which the barriers between the artist's work and his life were forever shifting and crumbling.

By this I don't just mean that art and life illuminate each other, which is an idea at least as old as Samuel Johnson's *Lives of the Poets* and too obvious to need arguing. For example, you can't properly understand Ezra Pound's *Cantos* until you take into account how the poet dealt with his enormous energy and talent in his life. The force he dissipated in sheer literary busyness – founding magazines, laying down the law, promoting other writers' work – then later dissipated again in political and economic paranoia – ranting away in defence of fascism and Social Credit – is somehow reflected in what was to have been his great work. The dispersal and deliquescence of the later Cantos is the aesthetic parallel of his own dottiness and fragmentation as a man. That idea is, as I say, self-evident.

What I mean is something more radical and confusing: the general belief – by the public as well as the artists – that the work and the life are not

only inextricable but also virtually indistinguishable. Out of this, something new and disturbing emerged during the '60s and '70s, and it is still
around in a debased form. I call it the myth of the artist and it is not,
believe me, what I had in mind when I wrote *The Savage God*.

Initially, the myth was based on the terrible precedent set by Sylvia
Plath, and the tragic way in which her life and her art complement each
other. Elizabeth Hardwick, who admires Plath's poetry and is appalled by
her story, has this to say: 'She, the poet, is frighteningly there all the time.
Orestes rages, but Aeschylus lives to be almost seventy. Sylvia Plath,
however, is both heroine and author; when the curtain goes down, it is her
own dead body there on the stage, sacrificed to her plot'.[4] Plath, of course,
was by no means the first important artist to die dramatically by her own
hand. Almost two hundred years before her, Chatterton committed suicide
and became, as a result, a great Romantic symbol. But at least he didn't
write about the act. Neither did Hemingway or Hart Crane or Randall
Jarrell or even, in so many words, Virginia Woolf. To follow the logic of
your art to its desolate end, as Sylvia Plath did, and thereby turn yourself
into the heroine of a myth you yourself have created was something
unprecedented. It changed the nature of the game. Art, that most stringent
and solitary of disciplines, suddenly came to resemble a high risk activity,
like sky-diving.

If nothing else, it was one in the eye for the Freudian theory of art as
compensation and self-therapy. Lawrence once wrote, 'One sheds one's
sicknesses in books – repeats and presents one's emotions to be master of
them'.[5] I myself believe that this is the exact opposite of the truth: you
don't shed your sicknesses, you dredge them up in writing and thereby
make them more readily available to you, so that you find yourself living
them out. Nature, that is, always imitates art, usually in a sloppy and exaggerated way.

John Berryman, for instance, began his great cycle of *The Dream Songs* as
a kind of poetic daybook, recording his gripes, hangovers, alcoholic guilt
and very occasional highs. Then he gradually deepened it into an extended
act of mourning for various friends tragically dead before their time. That,
in turn, led back to what was, for him, the primal suicide – that of his
father, who shot himself when Berryman was twelve. And so on, back and
back, deeper and deeper, until in the end – particularly in the beautiful
series of Dream Songs entitled 'Opus Posthumous' – he seemed to be
writing his own epitaph, as if there were no one else he could trust with the
job. At which point, the way was clear to take his own life. Which he did. It
seemed – perversity notwithstanding – the most logical means of completing his magnum opus.

That, anyway, is how the public seemed to read the story of Berryman's
desperate and messy last years. Portrait of the artist painting himself into a
corner. Portrait also of a situation which has got out of hand, for it is based

on a total misunderstanding of the nature of art. It is utterly untrue to believe that Extremist art, or any other art, has to be vindicated or justified by an extremist life, or that the artist's experience on the outer edge of the intolerable is in any way a substitute for creativity. In fact the opposite is true, as I have written elsewhere again and again: in order to make art out of deprivation and despair the artist needs proportionately rich internal resources and proportionately strict control of his medium. We have the Collected Works – or should that be the Collected Depression? – of Samuel Beckett to prove the point. An artist is what he is, not because he has lived a more dramatic life than other people but because his *inner* world is richer and more available, and also, more importantly, because he loves and understands whichever medium he uses – language, paint, music, film, stone – and wants to explore its possibilities and make of it something perfect. I think it was Camus who once remarked that Nietzsche's work proves that you can live a life of wildest adventure without ever leaving your desk. With all due deference to the late R. D. Laing, schizophrenia is not necessarily a state of grace and there are no short cuts to creative ability, not even through the psychiatric wards of the most progressive mental hospitals.

But schizophrenia, alas, is a good deal more common than creative ability, so it is not hard to understand why Laing's theories should have been so appealing, especially to the bards of the drug culture. What is baffling is that real poets should have gone along so readily with them. How else, for instance, to explain the astonishing lack of professionalism in Anne Sexton's books? Her trouble was not that she wrote bad poems, as every poet does from time to time, but that, instead of throwing them away, she printed them cheek-by-jowl with her purest work. The reason was that the bad poems were bad in much the same way as the good were good: in their head-on intimacy and their persistence in exploring whatever was most painful to her. She was unable to resist the temptation to draw attention to the raw material, as though whatever was sufficiently naked and overwhelming just couldn't fail. As Randall Jarrell once wrote in an essay about amateur verse, 'It is as if the writers had sent you their ripped-out arms and legs, with "This is a poem" scrawled on them in lipstick'.[6]

The truth is, great tragic poems are not necessarily inspired by great tragedies. On the contrary, they can be precipitated, like pearls, by the smallest irritants, provided the poet's secret, internal world is rich enough. William Empson once remarked that the opening line of Keats's 'Ode to Melancholy' – 'No, no; go not to Lethe; neither twist...' – 'tells you that somebody, or some force in the poet's mind, must have wanted to go to Lethe very much, if it took four negatives in the first line to stop them'.[7] By the same token, the more exposed and painful the theme, the more delicate and alert the artistic control needed to handle it. According to a psychoanalyst, Hanna Segal, there is one fundamental difference between the neurotic and the artist: the neurotic is at the mercy of his neurosis, whereas the artist, however neurotic he may be outside his work, has *in his capacity as an artist* a highly realistic understanding both of his inner world and of the techniques of his art.[8]

For example, Anne Sexton's good poems have an expressive tautness and inevitability in the rhythm which not only drives them forward but also keeps them whole. In her bad poems, the need to express gives way to an altogether less trustworthy inspiration: the sheer pleasure of confessing in public, of letting it all hang out, and you can hear it in the way the rhythm slackens and blurs into a kind of hypnotic chanting. What begin as real poems often end in an operatic no man's land, that shadow zone between Grand Opera and soap opera.

That in itself is nothing new. All sorts of talented writers have had their moments on the borderline of hysteria – Shelley, for instance, Lawrence, Dostoevsky. To lose one's poise is an occupational hazard for the experimental artist, trying to make it new. The specifically modern ingredient Anne Sexton and lesser poets added to the mixture was not that they occasionally lost control and thus become hysterical, but that they were hysterical *on purpose*.

This perhaps is the major danger of existential art. The theory can become a justification for letting go the art – by which I mean the solitary discipline and self-abnegation, the craftsman's patience and concentration in the face of his material. In the end, the poetry not only becomes indistinguishable from the psychopathology, it becomes secondary to it.

No doubt some of the blame lies with the media and their insatiable hunger for news. Art fashions may be news of a kind, but the scandalous lives of artists make much better news. 'Real art', said Susan Sontag 'has the capacity to make us nervous'.[9] Not so real artists, who tend to be battered, fallible, vain, and boringly self-centred. So by concentrating on them and their unspeakable lives, you can sidestep the effects of their art. Nearly everyone, for example, knows about Sylvia Plath's broken marriage and despair and suicide, but how many of the thousands who fervently study the intensely autobiographical *The Bell Jar* have ever bothered with her sardonic, demanding, unforgiving, yet curiously detached poems? Similarly, perhaps her husband Ted Hughes's *Birthday Letters* became a best-seller not because of the beauty and power of his language, but because people wanted the low-down on their marriage.

Unfortunately, the artists themselves have cooperated in this degradation. Writing is, after all, the most solitary of pursuits – a sedentary, middle-class occupation like psychoanalysis, though more lonely because you don't even get to see patients. So it is easy, in your lighthouse keeper's isolation, to be taken in by your own propaganda and begin to believe the myth you yourself have created. Moreover, fame is addictive, particularly if you practise a non-paying, minority art like poetry. I think it was Robert Frost who said, 'The trouble with poetry is, there's no money in it.' He meant, I assume, that the only rewards, apart from those of the art itself, are the most slippery ego gratifications: fame if you can get it, and, if you can't, notoriety, malice, backbiting and jostling for a place on the ladder. Whence the phenomenon of the stars of the poetry reading circuit who, like American presidential candidates or the sacrificial kings in Frazer's *The Golden Bough*, offer their persons, their bodies, to the masses, and simply use verse as an excuse for this strange, primitive, ritualistic exchange.

Ultimately, it is a form of sacrifice. The general public is not much interested in poetry, but it does have a taste for licensed buffoons, scapegoats and tragic heroes, or for a mixture of all three, such as Dylan Thomas. I wonder to what extent his so-called 'friends' and admiring, ox-eyed public secretly envied him his genius and therefore, encouraged him to drink himself to death in the name of good companionship and the Romantic idea of what a Bohemian poet's life should be like.

What, in all this, is the problem for the critic and the reader? In this age of public scandal and private psychoanalysis, T. S. Eliot's neoclassical solution convinces no one. Hence the sudden prurient interest in Eliot's anti-Semitism and Philip Larkin's emotionally loutish private life, as though they somehow cancelled out the poetry. Unless you do what the university theorists now do and simply use literature as an excuse for non-literary intellectual games, it is impossible to brush the personal elements under the carpet and pretend they don't exist. They do exist, inescapably, and the Extremist artists I'm talking about seemed determined that their audience should recognise this fact. Perhaps it was a way of insisting that what they were doing was deadly serious. Why else should they have been willing to pay such a high personal price? So in the purest writing of the 1960s and '70s, there was a curious two-way movement: the reader looked through the work to see the artist in all his or her misery, then out of it again to see just how perfect and detached and artistically self-contained the work was, how untroubled by the artist's nagging personal disasters.

This is what happens in Sylvia Plath's late poetry or in the novels of Jean Rhys, especially in her masterpiece, *Good Morning, Midnight*. Rhys's heroines move in an unremitting continuum of misery and drunkenness which, presented simply as such, would be not so much unbearable as merely boring. She redeemed it with her elegantly casual, pared-down prose and her unwavering determination to fix the emotions in observed detail. By underpinning all that wretchedness with the ordinary, indifferent business of living, she made it, in the end, sharper and more painful. The detachment necessary to write as well as she did reflected back on the quality of the emotion portrayed.

Coleridge described this process eloquently in the *Biographia Literaria*: 'himself meanwhile unparticipating in the passions, and actuated only by that pleasurable excitement, which had resulted from the energetic fervour of his own spirit in so vividly exhibiting what it had so accurately and profoundly contemplated.' From this came what he called 'the alienation, and, if I may hazard such an expression, the utter *aloofness* of the poet's own feelings, from those of which he is at once the painter and the analyst'.[10] Since Coleridge was writing about Shakespeare, the implication was that creative detachment of this order was the final criterion of great art.

It is not, alas, a criterion we seem to find particularly attractive at present. Even a poet as devoted and intellectually resolute and lavishly gifted as John Berryman flinched away from it. He once remarked, in a *Paris Review* interview, 'the artist is extremely lucky who is presented with the worst possible ordeal which will not actually kill him. At that point, he's in business'.[11] This, I suggest, is the old Romantic Agony buttressed by some peculiarly twentieth-century theories: a theory of existentialist aesthetics and a simplified psychoanalytic theory of the therapeutic relationship of art to life. If you think about this kind of statement, then remember how Berryman died, how Sylvia Plath died, how Anne Sexton died – all of them passionately believing that this was how the game was played – you have to conclude that no poetry, however fine, is worth the cost.

But there was another element involved, less tragic, less heroic: Berryman's remark, that is, was also influenced by his intense, competitive involvement with the media and with the idea of fame. Not long before he died, Berryman wrote an indifferent autobiographical novel about alcoholism, *Recovery*, whose polymath hero seems to embody all the author's most grandiose fantasies: he is Alan Severance M.D., Litt.D., a Professor of Immunology and Molecular Biology who also teaches a humanities course on the side. Like Berryman, Severance is an alcoholic who is being dried out. Like Berryman, too, he has been interviewed by *Time* and *Life* and simply can't get over it. Berryman has this to say of him: 'Severance was a conscientious man. He had really thought, off and on for twenty years, that it was his duty to drink, namely to sacrifice himself. He saw the products as worth it'.[12] As a rationale for alcoholism, this strikes me as being as fanciful and self-aggrandising as Severance himself and it becomes convincing only when you turn it inside out: given Berryman's belief in the connection between art and agony, given also the public's appetite for bad behaviour in its artists (which deflects it from the necessity of taking their work seriously), it may be that, for Berryman, the poetry became an excuse for his drinking.

At that point art itself becomes a sideshow of no genuine intrinsic value. All that matters is the disturbance from which art might emerge, given the right distraught talent and the right disastrous circumstances. In other words, the artists whom the '60s public found most alluring were those who knowingly cooperated in their own destruction. Having created myths of themselves as a by-product of creating art, they finished by sacrificing themselves to those essentially trivial myths.

Maybe this desperation was a reaction to something in the political air: the Cold War, McCarthy's witch hunts, the threat of nuclear holocaust and the war in Vietnam. Now times have changed, the stakes have got smaller, the arts are milder, less adventurous, less demanding, and Extremist poetry is no longer in fashion. Neither is its retarded sibling, Confessional verse, as promoted by Allen Ginsberg and the Beats, though it was they, in fact, who started us off on the melancholy road to what we have now: the artist as personality and performer, the artist whose ultimate work of art is himself or herself. For example, far more people know about Tracy Emin's shabby early life – the rape, the abortions, the boozing – than have ever seen even a reproduction of any of her work. Perhaps you might call this the ultimate free-market art-form: the artist's aim is no longer to create something perfect which, in Coleridge's words, 'does not contain in itself the reason why it is so and not otherwise';[13] it is, instead, to create a marketable personality that can be promoted on television and in the style sections of the Sunday supplements. As for Extremism, I wouldn't want all that trouble back, but the work that came out of it was great while it lasted.

Notes

1 T. S. Eliot, *The Criterion*, II.7 (April, 1924), 'A Commentary', p. 17.

2 T. E. Hulme, 'Romanticism and Classicism', *Speculations: Essays on Humanism and the Philosophy of Art (1924)*, ed. Herbert Read, 2nd edn (New York, 1936), p. 118

3 T. S. Eliot, 'Tradition and the Individual Talent', *Selected Essays*, 3rd edn (London, 1951), p. 21.

4 Elizabeth Hardwick, *Seduction and Betrayal: Women and Literature* (London, 1974), p. 107.

5 Aldous Huxley, ed., *The Letters of D. H. Lawrence* (London, 1932), p. ix.

6 Randall Jarrell, 'A Verse Chronicle', *Poetry and the Age* (London, 1955), p. 160.

7 William Empson, *Seven Types of Ambiguity*, 3rd edn (London, 1953), p. 205.

8 Hanna Segal, *The Work of Hanna Segal: A Kleinian Approach to Clinical Practice* (New York, 1981), p. 197.

9 Susan Sontag, *Against Interpretation and Other Essays* (New York, 1961), p. 96.

10 Samuel Taylor Coleridge, *Biographia Literaria*, ed. John Shawcross, 2 vols (Oxford, 1939), vol. 2, ch. 15, pp. 17–18.

11 George Plimpton, ed., *Writers at Work: The Paris Interviews*, Fourth Series (London, 1977), p. 322.

12 John Berryman, *Recovery* (London, 1973), p. 96.

13 Coleridge, *Biographia Literaria*, vol. 2, ch. 14, p. 9.

12
On Writing Madness

A. S. Byatt in conversation with Ignês Sodré

ASB Ignês and I met by accident almost. We didn't know each other and we were asked to talk as psychoanalyst and writer about the novel *Middlemarch*, with which we were both obsessed, and are still obsessed. And we didn't quite know what we had let ourselves in for, but we have been talking to each other as novelist and psychoanalyst ever since. When we talk I try to talk very much more as a writer, and I try to persuade Ignês, who is a very great reader, to talk professionally as an analyst – and you will observe that she slips in and out of these two hats. As indeed I do. We think up what we would like to talk about, and then we talk very much as we would talk to each other, with you eavesdropping – so it has a structure, but it's free at the same time. Today we are going to talk about the structure of Flaubert's *Madame Bovary* and Thomas Mann's *Death in Venice*, with excursions into other things. Ignês has written a very interesting paper on *Madame Bovary*, which starts with a reference to Freud's paper on creative writers and daydreaming. I shall start by asking her to speak about that.

IS Freud was a great reader of literature – including English literature; he thought that creative writers – and great artists – have a much greater access to the depths of the human mind than other people have, and that psychoanalysts can, and should, learn from them. Examples and quotations from Shakespeare are never far from his mind. He didn't write very much about creative writing. *Creative Writers And Daydreaming* was written in 1907, so it corresponds in time to Thomas Mann's *Death in Venice*, which is one of the works we are going to discuss. In this paper he compares children's play, daydreaming and the play of imagination, and tries to understand what happens when somebody actually writes a work of literature: how wishful thinking and fantasising come into it in the beginning, as well as experiences from the past. He is deeply interested in the process of transforming both real experience, and what in a way is the opposite of experience, wish-fulfilling fantasy, into material that can become a work of art. Freud was in awe of the secret, special capacity that only an artist has of transforming mental contents into a work of art that will have a powerful effect on other human beings. At the same time, he tries to place it in connection to normal development, and to explain it; his explanations can sound reductionist, because sometimes he wants to force what he can observe, and also what is difficult to understand, into his new revolutionary theories. He also says that the understanding of the function of fantasy in a person's development is tremendously important; daydreaming is conscious fantasy, but of course Freud's major contribution was the discovery and understanding of unconscious fantasy. The great artist has a greater capacity to tap into unconscious fantasy than ordinary mortals have, which accounts in part for the power of great art. Everybody fantasises, although this capacity, as we know, can be unhealthily inhibited; but when fantasies take over the mind in an over-powerful, over-luxuriant way, then this leads to neurosis or psychosis. This is the kind of fantasy we will discuss today in our two characters, Emma Bovary and Gustave von Aschenbach.

It is an essential part of sanity to have 'stories', which are ways of dealing with experience; and the creative writer can transform those into works of art, but individuals, ordinary people, just have them as part of their mental life – a subtext of fantasies is permanently around in the mind; you could say that madness happens when fantasy takes over and disconnects you from reality. It is important also to keep in mind that 'reality', from a psychoanalytic point of view, comprises both what is outside, the external reality, and also internal reality, psychic reality. Psychic reality can be thought about as differentiated from psychic unreality, internal falsehoods, and all that aims at obscuring who you are in your perception of yourself. So we chose *Madame Bovary* and *Death in Venice* because the main characters, of course, do get taken over by over-luxuriant fantasising, so they lose contact with reality (external and internal) and they can't process what is going on inside themselves; these are narratives about a descent into madness, but written by people who are very much in control over the narrative and over their minds. What both Flaubert and Mann are describing, in their brilliantly imaginative way, is the misuse of imagination. So we have the writer as a sane person who is well acquainted with madness, describing madness in fictional characters; in this case the madness caused by excessive daydreaming, fantasising gone crazy: that's why we chose our two characters.

ASB   I thought as you were speaking, Freud in his time manages to distinguish between male and female daydreaming. Male daydreaming, he says, is concerned with ambition, desired positions and achievements, the need for admiration. He says that women on the whole, owing to the circumstances in which they live, have primarily erotic daydreams, and in fact, of course, both our characters, both Gustave von Aschenbach in *Death in Venice*, and Emma Bovary, are driven ... – I was quite interested that Ignês said they were driven mad, because they were both people who certainly died of daydreaming, but they are not clinically insane.

IS   No, but they are clinically rather ill, nevertheless. The kind of pathology that Flaubert and Mann invented for their characters is very interesting for a psychoanalyst, because their characters are not, of course, completely mad, inasmuch as they have some notion of reality; but they do funny things in their minds with their notion of reality. Emma Bovary, just to feed her fantasies of being a romantic heroine of a beautiful medieval romance, incurs tremendous debts, debts that in fact in the end cause her death. She is seriously addicted to daydreaming, which is very much like an addiction to a drug, and it is precisely her disregard for reality, and contempt for reality, which eventually leads to her suicide. She is not mad to the point of not seeing reality: she doesn't have hallucinations, or full-blown delusions; but she hates reality and wants to triumph over it. And, of course, Aschenbach does something very much like that. In his mind he de-realises the plague which is taking over Venice, and the horrors of cholera; he is not mad in that he knows there is such a thing as cholera, in fact he sees decay everywhere in Venice – but this perception is kept in the part of his mind which is completely separate from the part of his mind where his infatuation with Tadzio is located. His relation with Tadzio is, of course, almost entirely imaginary. Both Emma and Aschenbach are mentally ill, but they are not clinically insane.

ASB   No. I think their dreams are very, very different in the objects to which they attach themselves. I see Emma Bovary's daydreams as partly a very cool cultural analysis by Flaubert of the kind of daydreams that a woman from a peasant background would have, a woman who had been sent to a convent and exposed to a kind of religious *schwärmerei*, and had then moved on to reading romantic novels and developed a vague imaginary world wrapped in beautiful veils and full of wonderful galloping horses and charming people seen at a distance. Flaubert makes the association of the reading of romantic novels with daydreaming, and also the association of religion with daydreaming. We haven't got time to go into it, but George Eliot's first review was written of a book by the French historians Michelet and Quinet, which was called *Priests, Women and Families*, and it argued that French men, with their erotic obsession, and customary separate lives with mistresses and male society, had allowed their women to have their children brought up by priests – in a sense as surrogate fathers. And the priests had thrust the children into a world of imaginary unreality – which is quite interesting, looking at it from a different angle. But you feel that Emma Bovary's inner mental life is consistently...

IS   ...consistently unreal, and her addiction to daydreaming distorts her capacity to face reality, which would be necessary to allow her to have some possibility of changing it. When she tries to do something to ameliorate her situation, she does it in pathetically absurd and ultimately destructive ways (for instance, in her attempts to transform her husband, Bovary, into a great and famous surgeon). Her efforts are not to do with effectively changing the world, but with de-realising it. She doesn't want to be a better version of herself – she wants to be a fictional character. She doesn't just want her fantasies to become reality, she wants to be fictional. She thinks 'I want to be one of those heroines of novels' – and she was a very bad reader, as you said. She reads good literature – she reads Walter Scott and she reads Balzac – but she reads it to extract props from it.

ASB She reads it to extract daydreams. She reads it to extract situations in which she feels better than she does in her own life – and has more status and better clothes. And I think the moment when we really realise just how unreal even her 'love' affairs are is when, after Flaubert's wonderful description of her first lovemaking with Rodolphe in the wood, after she has really committed adultery, because she finds her marriage so unsatisfying, she doesn't take it in until she gets herself into her bedroom and looks at herself in a mirror and says, 'I have a lover, I have a lover'. Which she says twice. And I think that's – it isn't the beginning of her madness because she's already been seriously depressed – but it isn't the same as actually loving somebody.

IS She doesn't say, 'I love Rodolphe, he's such a wonderful man'.

ASB And she doesn't even say, 'What a wonderful, passionate bodily experience'. She says 'I can now define myself a little bit: I have a lover'. And that is a daydream state of affairs. It's also normally human, I think.

IS But she overdoes it slightly, doesn't she? It is human, of course; what goes beyond the normal boundaries is how everything becomes exaggerated; she feels 'she was becoming, in reality, one of that gallery of fictional figures' – Flaubert puts it wonderfully, I think: to become, *in reality*, fictional... She thinks that she has now joined that 'lyrical legion of adulterous women'... – I don't know which 'legion' that was: I mean, there weren't so many books about adulterers that she could have read.

ASB I think it goes back to Tristan and Isolde. As Denis de Rougemont explained, the history of Romantic love in art and literature has been the history of adultery since the troubadours and the convention of courtly love for unattainable ladies. Lancelot and Guinevere, Tristan and Isolde are behind the longing for the forbidden which turns into the Romantic novel – more in Catholic Europe than in Protestant Britain. Wagner's *Tristan* was one of the great depictions of the entangling of Love and Death through impossibility. And Wagner's world lies behind Thomas Mann's.

IS I agree; but Emma Bovary has made the adulterers into legions: everything is very accentuated and made enormous. She is a hysteric. There is, for instance, a masterly description of her excited state of mind when she is in a coach on her way to meet her second lover, Leon, in Rouen: because she feels passionate, she imagines that a hundred and twenty thousand people, (this is *very* precise: the whole population of Rouen!) are sending her their passionate hearts, and her heart is inflated by a hundred and twenty thousand 'Rouenians' in love – so everything goes into a crescendo, and that's what Freud would think is over-luxuriant fantasy. It takes her mind over in a sort of frenzy, which is also what she needs to keep the passion going at its height, to make it 'real'. Emma's problem is that as soon as she starts losing the absolute intensity of her feelings, she starts descending again into discontent and eventually despair. This is why she is so severely addicted to a constant fictionalising of herself and of her life.

Perhaps we should move on to Aschenbach, who fictionalises one particular person.

ASB   His delusion does centre on a single person. He does actually fix his mind on an erotic object, which is a twelve-year-old boy on a beach, to whom he hardly speaks.

IS   He exchanges one smile with him. I think that's the only actual contact he has with him in the whole story.

ASB   And it changes his whole sense of himself. But if we look at the shape of the story, Aschenbach starts in a state of mind where he's ready to go mad, as you have said. The novel begins with a kind of dream vision of the world full of dangerous things. At the superficial level this causes him to think he should go on a holiday so he goes to Venice, where he falls in love with this dangerous, or perhaps not dangerous, boy.

IS   Thomas Mann imagines Aschenbach as a writer who in fact has written the same things Thomas Mann has written. It is as if he chooses a part of himself to be his hero. He starts with the problem of an excess of energy, threatening to get out of control: Aschenbach has to stop writing and go for a walk because his mind is going too fast. And then he starts seeing these uncanny, Mephistophelian people, or Dionysian people – grotesque, strange characters that frighten him.

ASB   It's quite interesting because he arranges all the people he sees into a kind of aesthetic pattern. He sees a strange man outside a small temple-like building whom he believes to be staring at him in a sinister way. As a literary device Mann intends his readers to make associations with the opening of Euripides' *Bacchae*, where the stranger god – who has come from the wild Orient (like the cholera in Venice, from steamy jungles) – appears on a hill outside a small temple, and threatens Pentheus. The suggestion of deformity and lameness does also recall Goethe's *Mephistopheles* – another supernatural personification of wildness and excess.

The whole description is too long to quote here, but this is part of it:

> ... and in his right hand [he had] an iron-pointed walking-stick which he had thrust slantwise into the ground, crossing his feet and leaning his hip against its handle. His head was held high, so that the Adam's apple stood out stark and bare on his lean neck where it rose from the open shirt; and there were two pronounced vertical furrows, strangely ill-matched to his turned-up nose, between the colourless red-lashed eyes with which he peered sharply into the distance. There was thus – and perhaps the raised point of vantage on which he stood contributed to this impression- an air of imperious survey, something bold or even wild about his posture; for whether it was because he was dazzled into a grimace by the setting sun or by reason of some permanent facial deformity, the fact was that his lips seemed to be too short and were completely retracted from his teeth, so that the latter showed white and long between them, bared to the gums.

When he gets to Venice he sees various sinister people on the boat and is taken out on to the bay by what he feels to be a sinister gondolier who might be simply taking him out into eternity; anybody with a classical education would immediately know that he is with Charon in a bark crossing the river into the land of the dead. His imagination connects the persons and makes them parts of a sinister threat. We are aware that Aschenbach, because he is so clever, is himself playing with this idea. We also know that Thomas Mann is playing with this idea – and played with it in life as well as in art. We know from the story of Mann's life that almost all the things that happen to Aschenbach did happen to Mann, and of course one of the terrifying things about madness is that everything in the world appears to be arranging itself around you, towards what is worrying you. This is both gleeful and terrible in this particular case.

IS This vision is not quite a dream, and it's not quite a daydream: it's somewhere in between. It is almost a hallucination – the content of which is powerfully visual, exotic, tropical, and erotic, with everything very luxuriant, and phallic, and rather vulgar and horrible too.

ASB Yes, it talks about hairy stumps thrusting up through boggy marshes and things like that. But also there are tigers lurking in this over-luxuriant jungle:

> His imagination, still not at rest from the morning's hours of work, shaped for itself a paradigm of all the wonders and terrors of the manifold earth, of all that it was now suddenly striving to envisage: he saw it, saw a landscape, a tropical swampland under a cloud-swollen sky, moist and lush and monstrous, a kind of primeval wilderness of islands,

morasses and muddy alluvial channels; far and wide around him he saw hairy palm trunks thrusting upwards from rank jungles of fern, from among thick fleshy plants in exuberant flower; saw strangely misshapen trees with roots that arched through the air before sinking into the ground or into stagnant, shadowy-green, where milk-white blossoms floated as big as plates, and among them exotic birds with grotesque beaks stood hunched in the shallow, their heads tilted motionlessly sideways; saw between the knotted stems of the bamboo thicket the glinting eyes of a crouching tiger; and his heart throbbed with terror and mysterious longing.

IS   Aschenbach is supposed to be a very intellectually severe writer, very much in control, who is suddenly psychically invaded by all this.

ASB   We have talked to each other about the absence of dreams, or even very coherent daydreams, from *Madame Bovary*, compared to the fact that Aschenbach does in fact have a dream.

IS   Yes, a real night dream.

ASB   How do you read the dream that we have here?

IS   The actual dream happens right at the end of the story when he is completely infatuated by this boy he keeps staring at; he feels completely compelled to look at him. He tries to leave Venice but somehow manages to be pulled back into it by losing his luggage:

That night he had a terrible dream, if dream is the right word for a bodily and mental experience which did indeed overtake him during deepest sleep, in complete independence of his will and with complete sensuous vividness ... the scene of the events was his own soul, and they irrupted into it from the outside, violently defeating his resistance – a profound, intellectual resistance – as they passed though him, and leaving his whole being, the culture of a lifetime, devastated and destroyed.

It began with fear, fear and joy and a horrified curiosity about what was to come. It was night, and his senses were alert; for from far off a hubbub was approaching, an uproar, a compendium of noise, a clangour and blare and dull thundering, yells of exultation and a particular howl with a long-drawn u at the end – all of it permeated and dominated by a terrible sound of flute music: by deep-warbling, infamously persistent, shamelessly clinging tones that bewitched the innermost heart. Yet he was aware of a word, an obscure word, but one that gave the name to what was coming: 'the stranger-god!' There was a glow of smoky fire: in it he could see a mountain landscape, like the mountains round his summer home. And in fragmented light from wooded heights, between tree trunks and mossy boulders, it came tumbling and whirring down: a human and animal swarm, a raging rout, flooding the slope with bodies, with flames, with tumult and frenzied dancing. Women, stumbling on the hide garments that fell to far about them from the waist, held up tambourines and moaned as they shook them above their thrown-back heads; they swung blazing torches, scattering the sparks, and brandished naked daggers; they carried snakes with flickering tongues which they had seized in the middle of the body, or they bore up their own breasts in both hands, shrieking as they did so. Men with horns over their brows, hairy-skinned and girdled with pelts, bowed their necks and threw up their arms and thighs, clanging brazen cymbals and beating a furious tattoo on drums, while smooth-skinned boys prodded goats with leafy staves, clinging to their horns and yelling with delight as the leaping beasts dragged them along. And the god's enthusiasts howled out the cry with the soft consonants and long-drawn-out final u, sweet and wild both at once, like no cry that was ever heard. Here it was raised, belled out into the air as by rutting stags, and there they threw it back with many voices, in ribald triumph, urging each other on with it to dancing and tossing of limbs, and never did it cease. But the deep, enticing flute music mingled irresistibly with everything. Was it not also enticing him, the dreamer who experienced all this while struggling not to, enticing him with shameless insistence to the feast and frenzy of the uttermost surrender? Great was his loathing, great his fear, honorable his effort of will to defend to the last what was his and protect it against the Stranger, against the enemy of the composed and dignified intellect. But the noise, the howling grew louder, with the echoing cliffs reiterating it: it increased beyond measure, swelled up to an enrapturing madness. Odours besieged the mind, the pungent reek of goats, the scent of panting bodies and an exhalation as of staling waters, with another smell too, that was familiar: that of wounds and wandering disease. His heart throbbed to the drumbeats, his brain whirled, a fury seized him, a blindness, a dizzying lust, and his soul craved to join the round-dance of the god. The obscene symbol, wooden and gigantic, was uncovered and raised aloft: and still more unbridled grew the howling of the rallying-cry. With foaming mouths they raged, they roused each other with lewd gestures and licentious hands, laughing and moaning they thrust the prods into each other's flesh and licked the blood from each other's limbs. But the dreamer now was with them and in them, he belonged to the stranger-god. Yes, they were himself when they flung themselves, tearing and slaying, on the animals and devoured steaming gobbets of flesh, they were himself as an orgy of limitless coupling, in homage to the god, began on the trampled, mossy ground. And his very soul savored the lascivious delirium of annihilation.

Out of this dream the stricken man woke unnerved, shattered and powerlessly enslaved to the daemon-god. He no longer feared the observant eyes of other people; whether he was exposing himself to their suspicions he no longer cared. In any case they were running away, leaving Venice... .

The dream is a lurid description of a Dionysiac orgy, and it ends with 'his very soul savoured the lascivious delirium of annihilation' – which points both to the horrible self-destructiveness which has taken Aschenbach over entirely, but also to a sense in which sexuality – this is more sexual fantasy than dream – is highjacked by what Freud later called the death instinct. When we discussed this passage before, I said that to a psychoanalyst this doesn't sound like a real dream because it's too much like the narrative of a mythological scene. And we both thought that it is too much like the Bacchae and the Dionysus story to be believable as the dream of an individual person, which would need to contain imagery that would be more specific to that particular individual. There is one moment only when the reality of present day Venice intrudes, when the smell of goats is mixed up with the smells of disease.

ASB   I think it's interesting how you – professionally – read the dream as a dream, before you read it culturally. It's a very, very ordered dream for a dream. And one thing it makes me think of is Freud's interpretation of one of the dreams of Descartes. Descartes had three dreams at a crisis in his life – in which he was haunted by phantoms, disabled and bent to the left, battered by a whirlwind and offered various things, including two books and a melon. Descartes insisted that these were dreams, not visions, and offered his own explanations. Later researchers wrote to Freud asking for his interpretation. Freud said in a letter to Maxime Leroy:

Our philosopher's dreams are what are known as 'dreams from above' (Traüme von oben). That is to say they are formulations of ideas which could have been created just as well in a waking state as during the state of sleep, and which have derived their content only in certain parts from mental states at a comparatively deep level. That is why these dreams offer for the most part a content which has an abstract, poetic or symbolic form.

Freud added that in his view the melon, which is not explained, is probably where a psychoanalyst would have something to say about what the dreamer was thinking about', i.e., the melon must have been the unconscious item. This is a great dream rather than a little anxiety dream, or repressed matter weaving its way up. This is a man understanding his situation by means of a dream – no?

IS   Yes, I think it is. Sometimes a particular dream is such a clear, meaningful metaphor for an important internal situation that it stays in the mind – this is clearly true of this Descartes dream (as we know, most dreams just naturally self-destruct). Freud did think that dreams contained elements of myth, and that the human mind contains primitive, powerful stories like myths. Well, he built a whole theory of human development based on the Oedipus story, so you can imagine how important myths were for him. Thomas Mann is clearly making use of a myth to create Aschenbach's dream: 'he thought the scene of the events was his own soul, and they erupted from the outside violently defeating his resistance, a profound intellectual resistance, as they passed through him, leaving his whole being, the culture of a lifetime, devastated and destroyed.' But this is also more than a dream, this is a picture of Aschenbach having a mental breakdown, and we thought that it was particularly interesting in terms of our theme of madness and creativity, because we see Thomas Mann at his most creative and sane and in control of his art, completely understanding somebody's madness, very specifically, that of a character created at least in part, and deliberately, after his own image. He describes his character's mind being totally taken over by his fantasies and by overwhelmingly primitive, uncontrollable impulses; Aschenbach is aware that he is losing control, in a way that is both terrifying and exciting, and you know that as the madness takes over he can only see this boy (the boy as he imagines him to be) and nothing else. In the story it is becoming more and more obvious that the plague is taking over Venice, so whoever stays there will die, but that has no reality for him any more, although he knows it perfectly well. So he is in the middle of this terrible destruction, but he is too overwhelmed by the process of his internal destruction to focus properly on what is external. Tadzio of course is not properly 'external' because Aschenbach is totally obsessed with a boy whom he has to some extent invented. So he has broken his connection to reality outside, and the connection to the reality of himself, even though he is never entirely deluded; external reality has lost meaning, the world and the people in it have become de-realised, although he can see that it all exists still. It is as if instead of having a dream, the dream has him: his unconscious fantasies, and his excited daydreams, have taken him over like a tidal wave.

ASB   Yes, that is exactly what happens to Aschenbach. We began by saying that this is about Thomas Mann being in control where Aschenbach wasn't. What Mann does, I think, all the way through *Death in Venice*, is to write very, very close to Nietzsche's book, *The Birth of Tragedy from the Spirit of Music*, where Nietzsche argues that Greek tragedy grew out of a Dionysiac orgy in which everybody became part of a group, had no individual identity, and in which creatures were torn to pieces living and were eaten bleeding – a kind of satirical goat dance. Nietzsche argues that the whole of the theatrical chorus comes out of this primitive joyful glee in destruction, and the God Dionysus was ritually dismembered and ritually reborn in this rite. The name of the god Dionysus in this aspect of himself is Zagreus, and Tadziu is usually described as having this name that ends in 'u' – 'u', which is being cried out by the group of children on the beach. And I think you can prove – though that's not what we are doing here now – that as Nietzsche goes through *The Birth of Tragedy* discussing the difference between the reason of the religion of Apollo and the unreason and violence and destruction and glee of the religion of Dionysus, so the same pendulum moves through *Death in Venice*, which doesn't mean that it isn't a perfectly good description of somebody collapsing.

Perhaps we should go on to Galton.

IS   Yes.

ASB   The next extract we wanted to discuss is actually something I wrote, in which Ignês developed a professional interest, which is quite alarming if you are a writer.

IS   When we were trying to choose what to bring as illustrations for this talk, we thought that Thomas Mann has a purpose in creating this particular dream because it functions on several different levels, the cultural as well as the psychological one of the character's madness. But as an analyst I couldn't believe that this could be a 'real' dream. Whereas I thought that the dream Antonia described in her novel *The Biographer's Tale* seemed to me very much like a dream I could have heard in the consulting room. In the novel, Galton is travelling in Africa, as the real Galton did, a very dangerous and very troublesome trip. He goes to Lake Ngami and he sees lots of corpses, people who have been attacked and massacred and murdered. He also sees women who are alive but whose feet have been cut off so that their ankle bracelets could be stolen. He looks at the victims of horrible torture, and he describes everything like a scientist or an anthropologist, quite coolly. He is just calmly observing and describing what he sees. He describes horrible tortures that children have gone through – children being burnt alive, and a child whose eyes are gouged out by some soldier.

ASB   Quite casually, he says.

IS   Quite casually, somebody just picks this child up and gouges the eyes out and throws the child down on the ground again; Galton witnesses completely monstrous things. And in the novel Galton is writing home, relating these real experiences, and he says, this happened, that happened, the torture happened – and continues, in the same breath after describing the burning of the children, as if this is an ordinary letter: 'Andersson desires to be particularly remembered to all. With my best love to all the family, relations and friends, collectively and individually, Ever affectly.

Yours, FG.' He is emotionally completely detached from this horrendous experience. So from my point of view as an analyst, or from that of any ordinary human being, he has done something really peculiar in his mind: he has this potentially overwhelming experience, you can hardly read it on the page, and he treats it as if it's a piece of scientific observation. Then he has his dream; and the dream is a creation of Antonia.

ASB   The dream is a lie.

IS   It's an invented dream.

ASB   He never in fact got to Lake Ngami at all, but...

IS   Yes, the whole thing is a fiction, isn't it?

ASB   This bit is, the bit before was true. All the descriptions of tortures are in Galton's real letters, and are quotations from them.

IS   Yes. So in the dream he says he sees all these bones, and he's so horrified by his dream that he says, 'I can hardly bring myself to describe it'. And then he thinks more about it, and says that perhaps he should describe it as a sort of cathartic experience. So he says there are bones all over the place and people who suffered horrible tortures; and then he says about his dream that 'My mind retches at it still', because in the dream parts of the body 'joined together in fantastic conjunctions'. Now, before that, what he says is that he sees these bones, and flesh starts growing on them in the most horrible way; so it's not a resurrection, but it's like a bringing to some sort of half life these bits of body which then start floating around in a horrific way: 'raw, slippery flesh, livid or freshly bleeding, hacked about and mauled, to which unspeakable things had been done'. (In a way we could link this with the hellish things that happen all around Aschenbach and Emma, when they are working frantically at de-realising reality: gruesome physical details abound, and surround them, and fill the reader's mind.) In Antonia's novel, after his cut off period (Galton uses 'scientification' defensively, as Aschenbach and Emma use eroticisation), Galton says, in relation to his dream, 'I had performed much butchery on beasts as a young man':

> But I can hardly believe that the horrible tortures, the ingenious mincing and carving up to which this mass of manhood had been subjected, came from my own subconscious. My mind retches at it still. Parts joined together in fantastic conjunctions – nipples with eye sockets, and other unspeakable concatenations – all in pain, in pain. I walked amongst them, trying to discern a whole man, and came upon a half-flayed severed head on a pole, out of which – I swear it – *my own eyes looked at me sorrowfully*: As if to say 'Why have you brought me to this pass?' These heaps of flesh were inanimate but not immobile.

Now, I think somebody real could have dreamt this dream, because I think this is exactly what the mind does. He had the experience, which is de-realised because he can't stand it, and his ego then defensively splits it in two; he keeps in his consciousness the scientific part of it, the cool obser-vation, and he represses – something Freud always talked about – and psychologically 'throws' somewhere else the pain and the horror of it all. And temporarily the traumatic experience is not his, emotionally his. Remember Beckett's play 'Not I'? The woman is on the dark stage, and all you can see is her mouth; she describes mad events and keeps saying – 'Not I, not I': that's what the mind unconsciously does. Emma disowns what frightens her; Aschenbach does that with the cholera. The mind has this unconscious mechanism of defence which says, 'not I, not mine' – it pro-jects the horror somewhere else. You know: 'I'm not the bad one, I don't contain these horrible experiences; they are out there, they are not mine; they belong to evil people – nothing to do with me.' When Galton dreams this dream – (and this is in fact what a dream is for, if you can cope with it: to digest the indigestible) – it all comes back from this 'not I' place, to 'me' again, and it assaults him. So for instance, the detail of 'My eyes look back at me', I find, from a psychoanalytic point of view, tremendously realistic as part of a dream a person in that situation could have dreamt: his eyes saw the horror, but then it is as if the eyes that saw have been psychologi-cally separated from him, have been thrown away. And then, through his dream, his eyes come back to him with the pain that he had been unable to feel. Galton's eyes look 'sorrowfully' – not only with sorrow for the suffer-ing people, but also because he knows that he has done something horrible to them, and to himself as a decent human being, by being so disconnected from them. So he also suffers the pain of guilt for not having sympathised with these people properly: this is what his dream-eyes accuse him of. So I leave it to you to say how you did that.

ASB It's interesting – it's some time since I wrote this, and when I re-read it I started remembering where I got it. I put it together because I felt that Galton must have been in the state of mind that Ignês has quite accurately diagnosed. He went scampering about Namibia like a kind of overgrown schoolboy, learning to ride on oxen and giving magical hats to local chief-tains, but he saw these horrors: he saw the men trying to staunch cut off feet by driving the stumps into sand. And he says one very revealing thing, when he goes home, which I do quote: when he got on the boat he slept the first good night of sleep he'd slept since he went there, and he hadn't realised how strained he had been. So I thought he knew really. And he was … Galton was an interesting man because he knew and didn't know about things like madness. He conducted an experiment on himself to see if he could make himself paranoid – which wasn't, I think, a word that then existed – by going through the streets of London supposing that everything was spying on him, until he couldn't stand going anywhere near a carriage horse because they made him so nervous. He decided he would learn how to worship a fetish, so he set up a picture of Mr Punch out of *Punch* magazine, and asked its opinion before doing everything. And after a bit he said he became really frightened of its eyes, you know, when he went into the room where he'd put this silly picture up. There was a dreadful period when he nearly killed himself by deciding he had to be in control of everything so he wouldn't breathe without being conscious of every breath, and he found that he just couldn't get the rhythm of his breathing together. So he was a dissociated person who was observing his own dissociation. But when I did the dream – what is really interesting is that Ignês brought up the idea of this dream, and I think you instinctively try to forget, as a writer, why you do something. I wrote the dream because I had thought for years and years about Thomas Mann and Nietzsche and the Dionysiac feast. This is actually my own conscious version of the cultural shock of dreaming Dionysiac dismemberment. Some of the things I put in I put in deliberately out of Lacanian criticism about *morcellement* – there's a psychoanalytical theory about the body snipped into very small morsels which occurs as a joke at the beginning of *The Biographer's Tale*. Lacanian theorists always quote a passage from Empedocles, Empedocles' image of the primal chaos: 'here sprang up many faces without necks, arms wandered without shoulders, unattached, and eyes strayed alone in need of foreheads.' So I actually dramatised that Lacanian observation from Empedocles in Galton's dream. When I put, for instance, the idea that the nipples were in the eye sockets, I was working off Magritte's surrealist painting of the woman's body as a face. So I was working quite consciously with material that is unconscious when you dream it. Having said all of which, I would like to say – which brings us onto the next part of our discussion really – that I threw myself into this dream as a writer by in a sense dreaming it. One thing I forgot, and should mention, is that Galton himself did actually have a sort of breakdown, during which he kept (he said) almost seeing a figure that he knew if he didn't make a great effort would appear on the wall of his bedroom, which was a crucified bleeding body simply pinned to the wall of his bedroom. He insists this had no religious significance: it was simply some body put up and crucified by the Roman soldiers. So what I did was to get all Galton's experience into my head, plus my own horror at reading his very cool descriptions of what had been done to those African women, and then I wrote the dream very fast, actually seeing it out of my eyes, and I didn't know until I got to the bit about his own eyes looking at him out of the half flayed head what I was going to do. But when I heard Ignês read out the word 'sorrowfully' I thought, of course, that's Christian: 'a man of sorrows, and acquainted with grief'. That word 'sorrowfully' is my (and Galton's) nod to, not the flayed God, but the crucified God; not the dismembered God but the other dying God who might be resurrected.

As is, of course ... you always forget the bit that really is closest to you: Galton quotes Ezekiel on the valley of dry bones that God allows ... God says 'shall these bones live', and they put flesh back on the bones, and the bones do live. That is my secret, most terrifying image of a novel gone wrong: a valley full of dry bones with the flesh half on, and the thing still can't get up and won't live. What you really want it to do is stand up and walk away looking proud and wonderful in the morning light, but you are dreadfully afraid that it will stay there with its bones and its flesh half alive, which is the most terrifying thing. And that's not Galton at all: that's me. So it's a sort of compressed amalgam.

IS   This is very interesting, as the fear of not being able to create 'new life' must be always there in the creative artist's mind – in your terrifying image of the novel 'gone wrong', of starting a process which will lead only to something destructive, 'with the flesh half on'; but in fact, as you say, in the writing this image is itself transformed into material which then becomes flesh properly alive, as Galton springs into very real fictional life.

But Galton himself must have been simultaneously very *un*-afraid of madness, to have wanted to make himself mad as an experiment, and in some other part of himself very afraid of it, otherwise he wouldn't be so curious about it. It seems to me that if you are going to be a creative writer (and since I'm not one I don't know, I'm just talking off the top of my head), you have to have a mind that you can use in a way not dissimilar from the way Galton uses his: I don't mean of course his defensive coldness, but the way that you have, rather bravely, to experiment with things, with strange states of mind: I imagine you have to sail very close to the wind. I think that's a link between 'madness and creativity'. Madness can be idealised, which I think is the notion of R. D. Laing and the anti-psychiatry movement, which you are interested in as a phenomenon of the sixties (which you are researching for your new novel); and of course the whole idea that poets are really mad, artists are really mad, which I completely disagree with. I think to create something you have to be at your sanest: that part of you is the part that creates. But you have to be able to have a mind that is able to contain difficult, disturbing experience – which may need to include the experience of madness, which is what Flaubert and Thomas Mann are doing, and you're doing when you talk about Galton. In other words, madness is not a wonderful thing to be emulated or idealised, but it is a thing you have to be acquainted with, because it's a part of your mind, it's a part of everybody's mind to some degree; psychoanalysts believe that to be able to create something anew, you also have to experience your own destructiveness. If you are going to create something new you've got to start, whether completely consciously or not, from re-imagining your own experience, but you have to 'dismember' it, tear it apart before you discover a way to re-integrate it into a different being. You know – to create a new whole, surely.

ASB   You do, yes, and you do little thought experiments, which is a term out of hard science, not out of psychological science; it's more like Galton. Another dreadful thing Galton did was trying to decide if he could read the newspaper under water and forgetting to come up for air, and some of the things I do to myself are a bit like that. You put yourself in a kind of imaginary mental situation and see what happens, and see if you can think your way through it.

I think we might spend the last few minutes we've got talking about how we think Thomas Mann and Flaubert felt their way in, because they did it very differently I think, and any good reader has to find a relationship, a way of thinking and feeling their way into the way the writer thought and felt their way into the character. The thing I forgot to say in my introduction is that Ignês and I are slightly heretical, I think, in that we do talk about characters in novels as though they were real people, which both in the profession of literary criticism and in the profession of psychoanalysis you are not supposed to do. But any reader and any writer must at that level experience them as real people or they're not doing it properly. If you don't suppose that Emma Bovary is real at all you are reading a very weird book. And equally if Flaubert didn't suppose she was real, it wouldn't work. But I do think, having said that, the ways in which my Galton, who is a fragment, and Flaubert's Madame Bovary and Thomas Mann's Aschenbach are real, are three very different ways: they're not the same.

IS   No: they're written in very different ways; it is not just that they are different characters; what you're saying is that the reader has very different experiences, not just of these characters, but of the actual process of reading and how experiences are built with words.

ASB   Yes, and this is because the distinction I would make between the Flaubert world and the Aschenbach world is that I can't bear being in the Flaubert world. I think I will try and describe this very simplistically. I read *Madame Bovary* at the age of seventeen, and it filled me with terror. I thought that if being a woman meant *that* I might as well die now. Ignês has kept quoting in our e-mails, that Emma Bovary says she wants either to die or go to Paris, and I very briefly felt that dying was the only way out of life, out of the awfulness of things, if you had to have or to be Madame Bovary. And I feel as a reader that the whole world of the novel is a projection of this awfulness, and that all that saves it is the extraordinary beauty, and precision, and wit of Flaubert's language. There isn't a nice person in the book; the world is the world of the mind of Madame Bovary in which everybody is trivial. It's also the world of a man who wrote a dictionary of received ideas, which amused him, but that's a defence against – like Galton's letter writing – it's a defence against terror. And I think this beautiful style, which Proust described as a kind of marble covering, is a defence against terror. Whereas I actually feel rather cheered up by the intelligence of Thomas Mann.

IS   Just going back for a minute to *Madame Bovary* – I think that's right: I think there is nothing felt to be of value; there is such contempt for everything. You quoted D. H. Lawrence saying, 'Flaubert treats reality as if it was leprosy', and I thought, this is very dramatic, but it is true in a way.

ASB   He said it in a review of *Death in Venice*, moreover, which is really interesting.

IS   Yes, which is really interesting – *Death in Venice* is about a kind of leprosy.

ASB   Lawrence says Mann and Flaubert resemble each other.

IS   In the two books we are discussing, there is a way in which they do convey a psychological situation about which they are both saying: if you have a mad relationship to beauty, if you cannot see both beauty and horror and find a way to integrate them in your vision of the world, if you feel you must keep your mind's eye only on beauty – beautiful boy, beautiful clothes, beautiful romance – something happens to horror, it doesn't just magically disappear; psychologically speaking, if you idealise physical beauty to the extent of isolating yourself from everything else that exists, then you will be surrounded by a world full of repulsive things, threatening to come back at you. And I think it is quite interesting how, in these completely different books, this is so clearly described. And in your book, this happens to Galton as well. Galton wasn't idealising beauty, but when he saw something that was unbearable, he idealised science and cold observation as a way of unconsciously protecting himself. The two books we chose are full of physical horror: horribly botched operations, diseased beggars, and the plague. Flaubert describes physical decay in absolutely horrible terms. Flaubert's father was a doctor, and as a child he actually saw corpses being dissected. Of course Flaubert and Mann are very different, and you would know much more than I do about literary criticism and their styles and their language, and the context they were writing in; but to me there is something that runs very close together, which is to do with authors who want to create a work of art which is a thing of beauty, and who are very preoccupied with the mind that splits beauty from horror, which they show as having terrible consequences.

ASB   Yes, these are both very, very self-conscious, very perfectionist artists who looked after every word, to whom their language was in a sense a justification for living, and I suppose Flaubert is more frightening because anything else in his world is more terrifying than anything else in Mann's world, which is full of ideas about the history of civilisation, some of which at least are interesting to think about, whereas the people in Flaubert's world only speak in dreadful clichés about nothing. They can't think, they don't care, and you are thrown back on caring about Flaubert's language. You were saying earlier that Freud, talking about daydreaming, very carefully analyses the structure of what he calls the popular novel – he says he daren't analyse the high literature novel – and he says that the popular novel is like people's fantasies in which there is *a* central hero and everything else is defined as either good or bad in relation to this person. There will be a shipwreck, there will be a battle: the person will survive. Every other character is either a helper or a demon or an enemy, and this is in fact a state of madness. It is also of course a state of affairs in every single fairy story I've ever read. There is either a male or a female central character, and there are things that help this person, and there are things that oppose it. And in a fairy story, as in a fantasy, it always comes out all right. But Freud also says that at the point where this gets really frightening you internalise your fantasy, and it becomes unconscious and then it can start tormenting you, and you see this happening to both our heroes.

IS   When the frightening fantasies come up in your dreams, in which case you can at least have some control over them because 'it's only a dream', you can also think about them; or at least the dream is a suitable place for them to be worked through. Or a creative writer can present transformations of those fantasies to you in a way that both enriches you but also helps you with working through them, not necessarily in a conscious way. But if fantasies so take over that they push reality away – the reality of who you are, fundamentally – then something destructive begins to happen.

ASB   And in that sense Madame Bovary was madder than Aschenbach, because he's got some sort of eye on his madness, and his dream tells him where he's got to. He's in a Dionysiac self-destructive mode.

IS   Thomas Mann wrote much more than Flaubert and created stories and novels populated with many, many characters; but if you think about the world of this particular story, *Death in Venice*, you only have in fact one 'real' character, Aschenbach. You have Tadzio, whom you never get to know except from the outside; in a way an imaginary character, a character in Aschenbach's imagination, who he wants to keep imagining, undisturbed by the constraints of reality. He doesn't, for instance, want to protect Tadzio from the cholera. He has death wishes in relation to him. He imagines him as Hyacinth, who dies, he imagines him as Narcissus, who dies. He wants to stop time.

ASB   Yes, and he finally sees him going out to sea, out into the 'misty inane', it says in the Lowe-Porter translation, out into, it says in German, the 'Grenzenlos', the thing without bounds, he loses form, he goes into the formless, i.e. death, or the unconscious.

IS   Yes, the underworld.

ASB   Tadzio is the psychopomp – the supernatural guide, often Hermes, who conducts souls to the world of the dead.

But then you come back again in a circle, having worked out that these characters are presented by their artists in a world in which all the objects the reader meets are symbols of the state of mind or state of psyche of these characters. Flaubert said that he wanted to tell the whole story with no metaphors but just things, and all the things in *Madame Bovary*, as well as being very real things, are things symbolic of her state of mind – boxes in which she gets shut, pointless objects she buys, like a prie-dieu, endless clothes which are somehow not clothes to put a body in but fetishised objects. And I don't know the answer to this question, but where is the reader in relation to a world, invented by an author, that represents, as it were, the fetishised state of the consciousness of a character? Some readers get deeply sorry for Emma Bovary, and some, like me, can hardly bear to remain in her company, because I'm so frightened.

IS   It's a horror story, really.

ASB   It's a horror story. But equally with Aschenbach, we know that Thomas Mann went to Venice and saw a beautiful boy, and we know that it's a revolving set of images. What Ignês has just said is absolutely right: we at no stage are allowed to meet any other consciousness than this consciousness that is constructing this world.

IS   Everything is unreal, and you only see it from the outside.

ASB   And yet what you are being given is not a fantasy entirely. It's a work of art, but it's a work of art constructed in the form of a fantasy.

The dialogue draws on the following works:

Beckett, Samuel, *Not I*, in *Ends and Odds: Plays and Sketches* (London, 1977).
Byatt, A. S., *The Biographer's Tale* (London, 2000, 2001).
Euripides, *Bacchae*, trans. Robert Bagg (New York, 1990).
Flaubert, Gustave, *Madame Bovary: Provincial Lives* (1857), trans. Geoffrey Wall, Penguin Classics (Harmondsworth, 1992).
Freud, Sigmund, 'Creative writers and daydreaming', *Standard Edition*, ed. and trans. James Strachey et al. (London, 1953–74), vol. 9, reprinted in David Lodge, ed., *Twentieth-Century Literary Criticism* (London, 1988).
Goethe, Johann Wolfgang von, *Faust*, 2 parts (1808 and 1832), trans. David Luke, World's Classics (Oxford, 1987 and 1994).
Laing, R. D., *The Divided Self* (Harmondsworth, 1971).
Lawrence, D. H., *A Selection from 'Phoenix'*, ed. A. A. H. Inglis (Harmondsworth, 1971).
Mann, Thomas, *Death in Venice* (1912), in *Death in Venice, Tristan, Tonio Kröger*, trans. H. T. Lowe-Porter, Penguin Classics (Harmondsworth, 1955).
Michelet, Jules, *Priests, Women and Families*, 2nd edn (London, 1846).

Nietzsche, *The Birth of Tragedy from the Spirit of Music* (1871), in *'The Birth of Tragedy'* *and 'The Genealogy of Morals'*, trans. Francis Golffing (New York, 1956).

Rougement, Denis de, *Love in the Western World* (1939), trans. Montgomery Belgion, revd edn (Princeton, 1983).

Sodré, Ignês, 'Death by Daydreaming: *Madame Bovary'*, in *Psychoanalysis and Culture: A Kleinian Perspective*, ed. D. Bell (London, 1999).

13

Breaking Down or Breaking Out?

Pat Barker in conversation with Adam Piette

PB   I should like to begin by reading two poems to you. One of the recurring themes in this essay collection is, 'What is the effect of a mental breakdown on creativity?', with the view being advocated that at least sometimes it enhances it. I want to read you part of a poem, 'The Rearguard', which was the first poem Siegfried Sassoon wrote after the events which led him to protest against the war.

> Tripping, he grabbed the wall, saw someone lie
> Humped at his feet half hidden by a rug,
> And stooped to give the sleeper's arm a tug.
> 'I'm looking for headquarters.' No reply.
> 'God blast your neck.' For days he'd had no sleep.
> 'Get up and guide me through this stinking place.'
> Savage, he kicked a soft unanswering heap,
> And flashed his beam across the livid face,
> Terribly glaring up, whose eyes yet wore
> Agony dying hard ten days before,
> And fists of fingers clutched a blackening wound.
> Alone, he staggered on until he found
> Dawn's ghost, that filtered down a shafted stair
> To the day's muttering creatures underground
> Who hear the boom of shells in muffled sound.
> At last, with sweat of horror in his hair,
> He climbed through darkness to the twilight air,
> Unloading hell behind him step by step.

And I also want to read one of the first poems Wilfred Owen wrote after arriving at Craiglockhart, where he had been sent because he was suffering from shellshock.

My lady owed a stripling lad
Unto her privie page.
Though five and ten he scantly had,
Both stalwarte was and sage,
And in his scarlette sylke y-clad
Was the flower of her equipage.

... But whan she conned she was overfond,
She sudden him dismissed,
Unto the Baron Oberond
She sent him all unkissed.

Well, as you can hear, it did nothing at all for Wilfred Owen's poetry to suffer from shellshock.

AP   I thought we would start with a remark that Rivers makes when he is thinking about treatment of trauma: he talks about medicine's 'split face'. He's been thinking about Sassoon's division, his dualism, and comes round to understanding that medicine may be similarly split, divided between emotional involvement in the patient and scientific objectivity.

PB   And he understands that both are essential: the doctor who is too involved burns out and is no use to anybody, and the doctor who becomes too detached from his patients ends up by just going through the motions. But, of course, the production of a war poem like 'In the Hindenburg line', for example, one of the poems Sassoon wrote immediately before coming to Craiglockhart war hospital, also requires of the writer both involvement and detachment. Sassoon had to be totally detached while he was re-writing the poem, but equally he could only produce the first draft by re-visiting the horror he felt at the time and re-immersing himself in it. So doctor and poet-patient share a particular need and dilemma, the balancing of these two forces.

AP   Would it be going too far to say that the cold-bloodedness of the craftsman – of the poet working the raw material of the war experience – is the same cold-bloodedness that Sassoon had as a commander in the field?

PB   It may be the same: in each case you are essentially exercising a craft, aren't you – leaving emotions out of it. I'm often asked, you see, whether a particular scene wasn't distressing to write, and I always say, 'Well yes, probably the first draft was, but by the fifth draft I wasn't feeling a thing'.

AP   Is there a kind of cruelty, therefore – in a broad sense, a necessary cruelty – in just this craftsmanship, after you've had the compassionate experience of, let's say, the first draft, the first imagining? Or a cool-headedness perhaps?

PB   Cool-headedness. There are writers, like Keith Douglas, for example, who actually aim to incorporate that coolness into the finished work as part of the artistic effect they're trying to create. Sometimes one feels uneasy, and it's the same kind of uneasiness, I think, as you feel when you're looking at photographs of war: you know perfectly well that the person who photographed this terrible scene was simultaneously thinking about perspective, composition, lights, which filter they should be using, and that can seem to be almost as much an atrocity as the scene they're recording. But most of us accept that war photographers have to be our eyes, to show us what's going on in war, because unless we *see* it we can't make the proper emotional response. And yet there's a perennial revulsion against the detachment needed to photograph people who are in pain, or dying. It's not an accident that we talk about gunmen and photographers 'shooting' somebody. There's a kind of aggression in pointing a camera at somebody in distress. We feel a revulsion from it and I think this is something war photographers themselves also feel. And there are cases when they go too far, and they're so keen on getting the photograph that they actually obstruct the rescue operation, or whatever. It's very rare but it does happen.

AP   Throughout your writing career you've taken a risk of another kind, in the sense of the tenaciousness with which you've kept to very dangerous topics.

PB   Yes. I admire quiet novels, but I don't so far seem to have succeeded in writing one.

AP   With regard to your work as a whole, I see three groups of novels: the first three – *Union Street*, *Blow Your House Down* and *Liza's England* – had a common concern with violence against women. And then you have the *Regeneration* trilogy and *The Man Who Wasn't There*, which move on to gender and war. And *Another Country* and *Border Crossing* are thinking about the family and traumatic issues. What links them, it seems to me, is the common concern with violence – would you accept that?

PB   With trauma and with violence.

AP   It seems to me it's trauma, but perhaps also something to do with coercive social groups.

PB   Even more than they are about trauma, I think they are about the process of recovery – and the process of defending your identity against the coercive and abusive groups, which in one way or another seek to diminish it. So I would always say that my books are about recovery. There's a much higher rate of recovery in my books than there is in life, believe me. In that sense they're optimistic.

AP   Does that optimism occur only at the very end of the books, because the working through and the working out is very, very dark?

PB   There are moments of illumination on the way, shall we say. *Border Crossing* is possibly the darkest book, in the sense that it doesn't end with anything much in the way of an unequivocal or unambiguous recovery. At least not for Danny. Tom is doing rather better than Danny by the end. On the other hand *Border Crossing* brings into play for the first time the idea that writing or other kinds of creativity are part of the process of recovery.

AP   Could we think a little about endings and the idea of the trilogy – you have said in interview that you started off by thinking the *Regeneration* Trilogy would be a one-book project.

PB   Yes I did, but I obviously couldn't give a satisfying ending to *Regeneration* because Sassoon is going back to the war, and he believes even more strongly than he did when he arrived in Craiglockhart that the war is unjust. And Rivers is going to have to go on treating patients, although he's come to question the whole business of treating patients in warfare and sending them back to the front. So in no way is the last chapter a conclusive ending. And having decided that there had to be two more books – there were always three, never two – I then had to re-write the final chapter, doing the opposite of what I was trying to do originally, and emphasising the uncertainty of the future.

AP   I see. Might that mean that *Border Crossing* might create its own trilogy some day?

PB   I think the problem is that no amount of further development could give Danny Miller a stable ending. His situation, living under an assumed identity, unable to make relationships with people, is intrinsically untenable, and will remain so.

AP   A common and difficult question is why British culture is so obsessed with the First World War. I suppose there's a different, though related, answer to the question in your case, and that it has something to do with Nicholas Abraham and Maria Torok's theory of transgenerational haunting: the idea that repressed secrets, according to their theory, are passed on from one generation to the next in encrypted form. Do you think the First World War has worked in that kind of traumatic secret way in British culture?

PB   First of all, let me say I think Britain dealt with the aftermath of the war rather well. War memorials, and Remembrance Sunday, and poppies are excellent, because they provide support to the individual grieving person and the individual grieving family, and you can contrast that with Germany where they didn't have any war memorials. What can it have been like to be a German widow, or a German orphan, with no sense of validation, no recognition of the importance of the life that was lost? I think what happened with the First World War is that in every generation we were prepared to emphasise some aspects of it and not the others. So that the initial memorials of the war tended to be quite militaristic: it was very much a matter of men parading with their medals on, and Geordie in *Another World* can't stand that, he just gets away from it. And then in the 1960s they were questioning the reasons the war had been fought. They wanted to focus on the horror. So Geordie suddenly finds himself in enormous demand, going around saying how absolutely terrible it was in the trenches. But there are still things that he can't say: he can't talk about class distinctions at the front; he can't talk about the disappointment when you came back home and found those class distinctions still in force. So the things he's allowed to say at every stage of his long life are quite different. And I think at the end of the last century, when there was a tremendous revival of interest in that war, it was partly that society needed to gather the threads together, just as an individual does in old age, or before they face up to some change in their life. But it was also, in an almost uncanny way, that we seemed to be starting to re-enact it. Suddenly Sarajevo was in the news, and it sent a shiver down my spine, and I'm sure not only mine, to realise that Sniper's Alley was the same street in which the Archduke Ferdinand was assassinated. That is absolutely incredible. And not only that, but the Bosnian Serbs, to whom Princip is an enormous hero, actually put concrete footsteps at the place where he was standing when he shot the Archduke, as a memorial to this great hero. And the Bosnian Muslims came along and dug the footsteps up again. This was in 1995. So you realise the extent to which that very complex and brutal war in the former Yugoslavia, which was being fought over land and territory and resources, was also being fought over memory. As I think a great many wars are fought, over memory. And François Mitterand chose to go to Sarajevo, at some considerable risk – because landing at Sarajevo airport was very dangerous – on the anniversary of the day the First World War broke out. He was appealing to people's memories of the First World War, and what it had meant to Europe. Whether he actually succeeded in communicating that to a generation which scarcely knows there was a First World War, I don't know. But at least he tried.

AP   And those enormous cemeteries – the Thiepval memorial for the unknown soldiers – do you think they played a double role, because they're actually working within European cultures, places where you can go and, let's say, find a mourning process which is at once public and private? Do you think they were political statements as well about what Europe should always remember?

PB   Yes, I think they were. And I think it's going to be very difficult as this century moves on and people look rather greedily at all that land. This is something that seems to haunt Julian Barnes – what happens when somebody says, 'Well, look, why don't we keep, say, Thiepval, and the Menin Gate, and perhaps one or two others and get rid of all the rest? What's the point? After all, we no longer visit the graves of people who died in the Napoleonic wars.' I think my answer would be that that war, and the camps of the Second World War, represent something so fundamental about human nature, and what we are capable of doing, that they are timeless – one of the very few human artefacts which are genuinely timeless.

AP   The atrocities that were going on, or the institutional violence, were on such a massive scale on those occasions, that the imagination could not understand their totality. One of the things that Siegfried Sassoon's protests implies is that there are people who are deliberately not allowing their imagination even to start to understand what's going on. But there is a real question about whether any soldier could understand the trench system.

PB   I think they probably couldn't. I think their world, as Wilfred Owen says, was 'but the trembling of a shell'. You saw at night in the trenches what a particular shell illuminated, which was a row of bleached sandbags, dug outs, your comrades in your platoon, and this whole hinterland of trenches, which was so complicated in places that people did sometimes, by mistake, end up in the other side's trench system. The individual soldier couldn't possibly understand that. And as for the mothers and fathers who were going on guided tours of the trenches specially dug in Hyde Park, which were nice clean comfortable trenches because you didn't want to worry their mothers; what could they possibly make of it? Owen was quite exceptional in the sense that he wrote the truth for his mother and he asked her to disseminate it. Not in any anti-war mood at that time, but simply wanting the people at home to know what the suffering at the front was, and wanting people like his cousin to volunteer and lend a helping hand.

AP   That difficulty in imagining where they actually were – because they were in this hellish environment which was so vast, extraordinarily vast, an empire or a labyrinth all on its own – makes it an extraordinary irony that Freudian psychoanalysis starts off then, during the war, and as a consequence with an impossible job to do. I mean, what he has to do, Rivers, as the first British Freudian, putting psychoanalysis into action, and popularising it in a way, putting it into practice under those conditions, is to do something absolutely impossible, isn't it?

PB   And something which Freud himself, of course, before the war, had not succeeded in envisaging. Rivers didn't find any evidence from his work at Craiglockhart, or indeed at Maghull, for sexual repression being in any sense at the bottom of these men's troubles. So in a sense the material was not particularly well adapted to a Freudian interpretation at all. Freud at that stage was an enemy citizen, and a lot of people would not consider, for example, the theory of the unconscious mind or the Oedipus complex, for that reason alone. It required a lot of moral courage to stick up for Freud in 1917, and if you did it at a congress of doctors you were very glad to be in uniform when you stood up and said, 'Let's listen to him, it might be true.' But I think, you know, Rivers was essentially an anthropologist. In his 1917 *Lancet* paper on Freud and the unconscious, he describes his interest in these issues as being very recent and temporary. Not only had he not practised medicine before the war but he had no intention of practising medicine after the war either. He was a very eccentric and temporary therapist.

AP   But he had been exposed to very bizarre sexual practices as an anthropologist.

PB   Yes, he certainly had, and in that sense I suspect he was rather more broad-minded than most people of his generation. He had a perspective on his own society which very few people indeed had. You know, it's difficult to speculate about Rivers because Rivers was possibly one of the most reticent men who has ever lived. His biographer, Richard Slobodin, says that it was like writing the biography of a little known ninth-century saint who had left no diary, and no personal letters. He was a great burner of papers. Wise man.

AP   Maybe we could move on to your Rivers, then, and your Rivers starts off with an idea about poetry and creativity when he's thinking about Owen and Sassoon.

PB   I think what he starts off with is a belief that traumatic experiences should be faced and articulated – not dwelt on obsessively, because that's going to the other extreme – but for part of every day, instead of trying insistently and compulsively to forget, you should sit down and deliberately remember. You shouldn't run away from memories. And I think he would have seen Siegfried Sassoon's poetry as a way of Sassoon performing that concentrated, controlled remembering. He would have thought that writing the poems was part of the reason Sassoon had emerged, by the time he got to Craiglockhart, out of the experience of battle relatively unscathed. Rivers had a great difficulty with poetry because Rivers had no visual memory, and it's difficult to appreciate poetry if you have no visual memory at all. I would like to say something about Rivers's loss of visual memory. If you all think about the room you sleep in, or your living room, most of you – perhaps all of you – will have no difficulty in visualising it. Rivers couldn't do that. He couldn't see his living room – couldn't visualise his environment – and this loss was something that started to happen to him at the age of five. He could remember the ground floor of the house he lived in when he was five, but he could not remember any of the upper rooms, and from then on until the end of his life he couldn't remember the interior of any building he'd been into, he couldn't visualise the faces of his friends, and so on: complete absence of visual memory. It is actually quite startling when you think what that would involve. First of all, how did he learn anatomy? I can only suppose that the method of teaching anatomy consisted of saying, there's a corpse, what's that part called? What does it do? What does it connect to? Because I just don't see how he could possibly have done it in any other way.

AP   William Empson said he couldn't visualise either, and wondered whether that's why his poems were so rational, as if to say, 'I sound like Donne, because an image isn't an image to me: it's a sequence of words, it's an argument.'

PB   It would be difficult to appreciate Siegfried Sassoon's poetry with no powers of visualisation. Because it's one image piled on another. That's the way he works: he piles up photographic images.

AP   Yes. Jon Silkin has this very odd argument about Sassoon, that he couldn't regenerate himself because he had this passive visualisation, he was just a receiver of mental images.

PB   I think that's a perceptive observation. It's also what one feels about photographs – that a photograph can't tell you what to think, can't tell you what to feel. You are too passive in relation to a photograph to be able to utilise it fully perhaps. It's not interpreted for you enough, as a painting's interpreted.

AP   In terms of the dynamics of the novel, if Sassoon's the visualiser, and Rivers has censored his visual memory, it's Prior who really triggers Rivers' visualisation, though it's the example of Sassoon which makes Rivers courageous enough to go back into this extraordinary process of self-analysis –

PB   – that he goes through in the book. He also went through it, of course, in life. He repeatedly tried to analyse himself and recover the repressed memory that he believed lay at the root of his loss of his visual memory, and as far as I know he never did, and he would never use hypnosis to do it. So at least he was consistent: he wouldn't use hypnosis on his patients and he certainly wasn't going to let anybody else loose on his mind. I suggest that there's a possible source in the man who killed the man who killed Lord Nelson, his ancestor who had his legs amputated on board the Victory, which was an unpleasant process – no anaesthetic and they sealed the wound by pouring boiling tar over it.

AP   Yes, and it's very strangely related to the Lewis Carroll anxieties about being a boy?

PB   Yes. The friendship of the Rivers family with Lewis Carroll was a gift to me as a novelist. He became very fond of Rivers' little sister Kathleen, as was his wont, and rather ignored the two boys, William and Charles. You remember in *Alice in Wonderland*, Alice solves her problems – and sometimes creates others – by changing her body. That is very like the kind of hysteria Rivers encountered in some of his patients. Faced with the intolerable pressure to go on fighting, some men developed paralysis, contractures, blindness, deafness – so that it became physically impossible for them to go on fighting. It was a form of body protest against the war.

AP   The books are about gender because they're concerned with the way the very idea of masculinity is turned on its head by shellshock, male hysteria. You go beyond, I think, many of the feminists' point of view, in particular Elaine Showalter's point of view, in thinking of male hysteria as a symptom not only of the disintegrating and traumatic war experience of the individual soldier but of the nation as well – there was a kind of hysteria at the national level.

PB   Yes, I think there was. And it went on after the war. There's a very interesting unpublished and unfinished paper by Rivers in which he talks about the atmosphere of the post-war world and compares it with the processes an individual patient goes through after a traumatic shock: the numbness, the denial, the frantic attempts to distract oneself from memory of the horror. And he could see all this going on around him and his undergraduate students in Cambridge after the end of the First World War. It's a pity it was never published. It's a fascinating paper.

AP   The Bloomsbury intellectuals are interested in shellshock in a very coded way, I mean, T. S. Eliot writes that little prose poem about hysteria, and Virginia Woolf has Septimus Smith –

PB   – who was allegedly based on Siegfried Sassoon. She identifies the emotional repression of the war years as the cause of Septimus Smith's breakdown.

AP   Yes, the S. S. of the names is the allusion. For both Eliot and Woolf, there's a comic and an anxious idea that the hysteria has some relationship to modernist creativity.

PB   I just wonder on the personal level what Virginia Woolf actually thought about it. It's very difficult to know because she writes so little about her own mental illness, and never in any detail, but it's always struck me as quite strange that one of her psychiatrists, one of the many, was Henry Head, a great friend of Rivers, who was himself involved in treating hysteria in soldiers during the First World War.

AP   Thinking about Henry Head, it is very striking that Rivers' neurological work – because we're thinking about self-analysis – is also based on the very strange experiments that Rivers and Head conducted.

PB   They cut a nerve in Head's arm and traced the process of regeneration over a period of four years.

AP   It's an odd probing of the unconscious, in that sense, because their idea was that the deeper you go into the body, into the skin, the deeper you are going back into the primitive.

PB   Yes, there is the idea that there were two layers of the nervous system: a protopathic layer, which was a very primitive layer characterised by all-or-nothing sensations; and the epicritic layer, which was more capable of making fine distinctions; and they generalised from that to psychological characteristics – epicritic criticism, conscientiousness, spirituality, etc., and the protopathic beast below. But what was interesting about Rivers was that he came to see the protopathic as a positive force and the source of a great deal of creativity, which I think also corresponds with his growing respect for some of the preliterate societies outside Europe.

AP   And would he have believed that the poetry that Sassoon and Owen were writing had a kind of direct line back to this primitive, protopathic dream-like or mythological power?

PB   I don't know that he would have associated poetry with the protopathic but he certainly would have associated it with dreams. He was fascinated by the links between poetry and dreams and the myths of primitive peoples, and the way in which symbolism is used in these three fields. He was fascinated by dreams partly because of Freud's idea that they were the window into the unconscious, but also for the very personal reason that he recovered his powers of visualisation in his dreams.

AP   Would you see yourself as a scientific, controlling and experimenting novelist? On Radio 4, you said you prefer that model of the writer to the idea of the writer as some confabulating mental health patient, as it were.

PB   I don't think that fiction writing and the delusions of certain forms of mental illness have very much in common at all. We do know what writers suffer from: chronic mild depression, with a strong tendency to self-medicate on alcohol. Hemingway says that the essential piece of equipment for a writer of fiction is a built-in, shockproof bullshit detector. There is an argument that the mildly depressed actually have a more objectively valid view of themselves and their situation than the people who go through life feeling fairly cheerful. It could be argued that what we all need is a slight dose of delusional thinking, and that writers of fiction tend not to have enough of it.

AP   So you wouldn't see an analogy between the way your fiction writing deals with very painful areas of experience – national, cultural, private – and what Head and Rivers went through in that extraordinary, experimental self-mutilation for science.

PB   Yes, I think perhaps so. You set up a fictional world, and you work out what the rules of the fictional world are, and what happens if somebody tries to disobey those rules. It doesn't have to be realist fiction of course. If you were Tolkien you might ask, what would happen to an Orc who objected to killing Hobbits. It is this very deep sense of what the possibilities are, and if you are going to suggest that something extraordinary can happen then you have to prove that it can happen in terms of the rules of the world you've set up.

AP   There are extraordinary things that happen and we are convinced that they happen in your books. Two of the extraordinary things that happen I think are the characters of Prior and Danny – Prior in particular, that uncanny way he has of being more powerfully an analyst than Rivers. We tend to talk lamely about people gifted with X-ray vision, but he really has that, and it's what makes the encounters so powerful – the dialogues of Prior with Rivers and others are some of the most powerful things you've written.

PB   And of course Prior is continually learning from Rivers. If you've got somebody, shall we say with a troublesome personality, and you subject them to psychotherapy the only certain outcome is that they will learn the techniques of psychotherapy, and because these techniques are powerful, if they were dangerous and troublesome before, they will be more so by the time you've finished with them. You may also, of course, be doing some good, but that isn't an inevitable outcome. Whereas the patient's learning the techniques of therapy is.

AP   It is a process of possession, appropriation and telepathy, I mean, his power to intuit goes beyond simply canny, streetwise, fly knowingness.

PB   Yes, he has extraordinary empathy. He has empathy without compassion. Now that is a very frightening thing. Rivers has both.

AP   One of the things I don't think your novels do is suggest that there is a sort of direct cause for extraordinary personalities like Prior. One of the questions that goes through the reader's mind is whether Prior is a product of a battle of the sexes, which is another kind of war occurring at the same time as the First World War. Prior himself talks about 'he and she', elemental forces 'clawing each other in every cell of his body'. Would it be true or unwise to say that it was the battle of the sexes in its nightmarish forms which formed the hinterland to personalities like Prior and Danny?

PB Yes, I think in a way they are both products of a very firm identification with mothers who were not capable of standing up at all to
violent fathers, and that there is both a very powerful identification with
the mother but also a contempt for her because she can't handle the situation, a feeling of betrayal because she doesn't protect the child. Yes, they
do have a lot in common. Sexual ambiguity, a capacity for violence – I'm
not making, for heaven's sake, any kind of general point about men,
because this is a very unusual personality structure. People often ask how
far do you as novelist use real people as the basis for a character. One of the
originals for Danny Miller was a journalist who interviewed me about
Another World. He introduced himself by saying he had a diagnosis of
severe borderline personality disorder and that was why he was so good at
his job, because it gave him an unusual capacity for empathy. And I
thought, I don't believe that: there's no personality disorder which
enhances empathic abilities. What he actually had was an inability to
recognise where he stopped and other people started, so he would attribute
his views to the person he was interviewing – and do so in all sincerity. I
was fascinated – both by the fluidity of his identity, and by the way he had
incorporated the diagnosis until it had become the crucial fact about him –
but given it a positive gloss, too, so he was able to live with it. As I say, he
was one of the originals for Danny, but of course the reason I was so struck
by him was that he reminded me of my own character Billy Prior. I don't
want to imply that Danny Miller and Billy Prior are the same character
because they are certainly not. You put Danny Miller alone in a room, the
room is empty. You put Billy Prior alone in a room, it rapidly becomes
overcrowded. There are very different things going on inside those two,
and there's a hollowness in Danny Miller which isn't there in Prior.

AP Yes, but there is one common thread between the two characters,
which is war, in the sense that there's a kind of training through the
father's violence into an extraordinarily perverse idea of the military ethic,
or perhaps it is the military ethic as such?

PB Danny Miller's father has categories of people whom it's permissible
to kill: enemy soldiers, people who you have good reason to suspect of
being terrorists, and all these concentric circles of who can be killed and
who can't be killed, which makes him sound terribly abnormal, except that
his concentric circles are exactly the same as ours. He's voicing the values
of mainstream society.

AP But might this still relate to the war zones of modern life which you
identify to a certain extent with run-down housing estates and warrior
males? You talk about the warrior mentality, the warrior morality.

PB Feral boys really, yes. I think when you talk about a warrior mentality,
you are talking about young men who are economically inactive in their

communities, not responsible for rearing any children they may happen to have. They're very touchy about their personal reputation, they centre their idea of themselves as men on being very tough, physically brave rather than on being reliable and valuing the things that perhaps a more mature man might focus his attention on. To what extent is this like soldiers? I don't think it's very like soldiers at all. I think the typical warrior in the First World War was Siegfried Sassoon, who was incredibly brave, and he was still a second lieutenant in 1917, because it took a lot more to be an officer than simply being brave. In fact the standard manual issued to officers actually discourages company commanders from displays of personal courage. They were irrelevant. But, of course, if you're a warrior they're not irrelevant. If you're a warrior, displaying personal courage and acquiring a reputation for toughness is precisely what it's about.

AP   So you'd say that that warrior morality is a kind of primitive drive rather than characteristic of the modern soldier?

PB   It's a very primitive thing, yes. And the professional modern army wants no truck with it at all. They want you to put the group first and keep your head down and avoid becoming a dead hero.

AP   Just thinking a little bit about your views on the modern nuclear family, there is an idea that when the family breaks down, becomes dysfunctional, it is a symptom perhaps of what has happened to the family in the twentieth century – that it has become too isolated from community, and within the hot-house of that family, love is too intense and authority can tend to be too focused, too sharply focused by this small conjugal unit. So that the breakdown tends to be almost immediately pathological.

PB   Yes, except that the modern family in *Another World* almost eerily replicates the Edwardian society where the marriage was broken and children lost their parents through death rather than through divorce. But it was still not unusual to have second or even third marriages and each of them would produce children. So you had complex but larger families less isolated than ours because, in the middle classes, there were servants in the house and, in the working classes, you had these very close-knit communities. The modern family can be very isolated. The tendency is to have fewer children, and to focus all the family's hopes, all its energy, in the children, who are very protected. At the same time the children on the local housing estate may be very much feared. I do see a kind of pattern of overprotection of one's own children, and the projection of quite negative emotions onto the children of the poor. I think our nervousness about children is essentially a fear of the future. And the children in our midst are the natural representatives of that future, and a lot of that fear is projected onto them.

AP   Do you think that it's time to revise the idea of the family? Because the family tends to be self-reproducing in more and more neurotic ways, if you think about familial protectiveness as really just fear.

PB   And therapists deal with the child in the context of the family, which is reasonable enough, but that's partly because the family is a unit small enough and powerless enough to be stigmatised. You don't see a child being dealt with in the context of a failing school or a failing community, though the problems of a particular child may derive from that just as much as from its own family.

AP   There's an extraordinary idea of time in your books and you think about time as viscous, unpredictable, like blood, and that it is like blood because it coagulates and clots around particularly dark secrets and traumatic events. And you have advocated, I think quite strongly, that, particularly in clinical conditions, one ought not always to feel that going back into the past to discover those dark secrets, those dark scars, is the only way we can do therapy.

PB   Yes. It's not the only way people do therapy. Many therapists take the present problem and focus very narrowly and very specifically on solving the problem that's bothering the client at the moment, and never mind how they got it. It's the problem of when focusing on the memory of traumatic events becomes counter-productive. It's true of societies as well. When I give readings in Germany, one of the things they keep asking is: 'Isn't there a wisdom in forgetting? When can we forget? When can we stop remembering these appalling things that have happened?' The ending of *Another World* is partly an attempt to get an answer to that. There is a wisdom in forgetting as well as in remembering, but the paradox of the memorial, and the special day is that they give you permission to forget, enough to get on with your life, because if you don't have memorials, and you don't have special days on which you remember, the danger is that your whole life will be swamped by grief. So remembering and forgetting go together.

The dialogue draws on the following works:

Abraham, Nicolas and Torok, Maria, *The Shell and the Kernel*, vol. 1, ed., trans., and intro. Nicholas T. Rand (Chicago, 1994).
Barker, Pat, *Another World* (London, 1998).
——, *Blow Your House Down* (London, 1984).
——, *Border Crossing* (London, 2001).
——, *Liza's England* (London, 1986).
——, *The Eye in the Door* (London, 1993).
——, *The Ghost Road* (London, 1995).
——, *The Man Who Wasn't There* (London, 1989).
——, *Regeneration* (London, 1992).
——, *Union Street* (London, 1982).

Douglas, Keith, *The Complete Poems,* ed. Desmond Graham (Oxford, 1978).

Empson, William, *Argufying: Essays on Literature and Culture,* ed. John Haffenden (London, 1987).

Head, Henry and Rivers, W. H. R., *Studies in Neurology* (London, 1920).

Owen, Wilfred, *The Complete Poems and Fragments,* ed. Jon Stallworthy, 2 vols (London, 1983).

——, *Selected Letters,* ed. John Bell (Oxford, 1985).

Piette, Adam, *Imagination at War: British Fiction and Poetry 1939–1945* (London, 1995).

——, *Remembering the Sound of Words: Mallarme, Proust, Joyce, Beckett* (London, 1996).

Rivers, W. H. R., *Instinct and the Unconscious: A Contribution to a Biological Theory of the Psycho-neuroses* (Cambridge, 1920).

——, *History and Ethnology* (New York, Toronto, 1922).

——, *Psychology and Politics: and Other Essays* (London, 1923).

——, *Conflict and Dream* (London, 1923).

——, *Medicine, Magic and Religion: The FitzPatrick Lectures delivered before the Royal College of Physicians of London in 1915 and 1916* (London, 1924).

——, *Social Organization* (London, 1924).

——, *Kinship and Social Organisation; together with The Genealogical Method of Anthropological Enquiry* (London, 1968).

Sassoon, Siegfried, *Collected Poems, 1908–1956* (London, 1961).

——, *The Complete Memoirs of George Sherston* (London, 1937).

Showalter, Elaine, *The Female Malady: Women, Madness and English Culture, 1830–1980* (London, 1987).

Silkin, Jon, *Out of Battle: The Poetry of the Great War* (Oxford, 1972).

Slobodin, Richard, *W. H. R. Rivers: Pioneer Anthropologist, Psychiatrist of the Ghost Road* (Gloucester, 1997).

Index